SOCIOLOGY OF HEALTH
AND HEAL

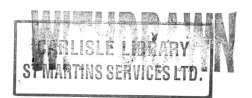

SOCIOLOGY OF HEALTH AND HEALTH CARE

Third Edition

Edited by

Steve Taylor, *BA, LLB, MPhil, PhD*
Senior Lecturer
The London School of Economics and *Coventry University*

David Field, *BA, MA, AM, PhD*
Visiting Professor
Department of Epidemiology and Public Health,
University of Leicester

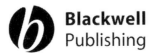

© S. Taylor & D. Field 2003

Blackwell Publishing Ltd
Editorial offices:
Blackwell Publishing Ltd, 9600 Garsington Road, Oxford OX4 2DQ, UK
   Tel: +44 (0)1865 776868
Blackwell Publishing Inc., 350 Main Street, Malden, MA 02148-5020, USA
   Tel: +1 781 388 8250
Blackwell Publishing Asia Pty, 550 Swanston Street, Carlton, Victoria 3053, Australia
   Tel: +61 (0)3 8359 1011

The right of the Authors to be identified as the Author of this Work has been asserted in
accordance with the Copyright, Designs and Patents Act 1988.

First edition published 1993 by Blackwell Science Ltd
Reprinted 1994, 1995
Second Edition published 1997
Reprinted 1999, 2000, 2001
Third edition published 2003
Reprinted 2004, 2005

Library of Congress Cataloging-in-Publication Data
Sociology of health and health care/[edited by] Taylor & Field.—3rd ed.
    p.; cm.
Includes bibliographical references and index.
   ISBN 1-4051-0869-X (pbk)
   1. Social medicine—Great Britain. 2. Social medicine. 3. Nursing—Social aspects.
4. Nursing—Social aspects—Great Britain.
   [DNLM: 1. Great Britain. National Health Service. 2. Delivery of Health Care—Great Britain.
   3. Sociology, Medical—Great Britain. 4. State Medicine—Great Britain. W 84
FA1 S67 2003] I. Taylor, Steve (Steve D.) II. Field, David, 1942–

RA418.3.G7S636 2003.
306.4′61′0941—dc21

2003000673

ISBN-10: 1-4051-0869-X
ISBN-13: 978-14051-0869-0

A catalogue record for this title is available from the British Library

Set in 10/12.5pt Century Book
by DP Photosetting, Aylesbury, Bucks
Printed and bound by Replika Press Pvt. Ltd, India

The publisher's policy is to use permanent paper from mills that operate a sustainable
forestry policy, and which has been manufactured from pulp processed using acid-free and
elementary chlorine-free practices. Furthermore, the publisher ensures that the text paper
and cover board used have met acceptable environmental accreditation standards.

For further information on Blackwell Publishing, visit our website:
www.blackwellnursing.com

Contents

Foreword

Since the last edition of this book in 1997, the delivery and organisation of health care has developed at a breathtaking pace. Health care reform in the United Kingdom, currently focused on a framework of centrally controlled targets and audit, has attracted much resistance and criticism from both health professionals and the public. It is my belief that future analysis of this period in health care history will identify this framework as a necessary and enabling intervention to move health delivery forward and away from the model that was right and appropriate for the post war society of the 1940s.

In 2003, health care delivery requires real and demonstrable accountability from all health care workers and the central participation of patients in the delivery and organisational structures of care. Successful health care depends not only on the clinical competence of staff but also on the organisation and structure of where health care takes place. The issues of pay, power and participation will, without doubt, be of concern to nurses, the hundreds of different categories of staff that make up the national health service and the receiving and participating public over the next 3–4 years.

It is interesting to observe the development of nursing at this time. Increasingly politicians are finding that health problems have nursing solutions. This in turn represents a constant and observable challenge to the past order of health care. Whilst it is accurate to say that nursing is emerging with ideas and adaptability that credit the profession, this is not without some painful and polarised 'old order' versus 'new order' political debate and manoeuvring. This professional evolution requires some tough 'out of the box' thinking that puts historical reference points to one side. Only then can nursing enter an historically exciting era that redefines this significant workforce in terms of the work of women and their professional organisation.

For future generations of nurses and other health professionals, sociological understanding of health care delivery and history is non-optional. This third edition of *Sociology of Health and Health Care* offers access to that understanding and is as fresh and relevant as the two previous editions. The additional three chapters give the reader sociological analysis of contemporary health issues and the whole text facilitates understanding and learning that enable the reader to experience and develop sociological thought.

Steve Taylor and David Field have produced a text that is essential reading for all health care students. Students will be both informed and challenged on their journey through these chapters. Discovery of ideas about care surveillance as a form of social control and patient information as a key factor in the balance of power between patient and professional, is sure to stimulate that 'out of the box' thinking that contemporary health care deserves and demands.

Roz Osborne *MA, BA, RN*
Director of Human Resources
North Hampshire Hospital Trust

Preface

This third edition of *Sociology of Health and Health Care*, like its predecessors, aims to provide a clear, easy-to-understand introduction to the area. As in the previous editions, the book is organised to provide continuity between chapters whilst also allowing each chapter to be read on its own. Although we have oriented the text and examples towards nursing, the book will also be relevant to students in other health professions. In response to requests and suggestions from teachers and the changed political context we have altered the structure and contents of the book in a number of ways, including introducing a new section on the social patterning of health and disease.

The introductory section has been revised and reorganised. Chapter 1, introducing readers to sociology, has been extended to include further discussion of sociological theory, research methods and the relation between them. Chapter 2, incorporating material from Chapters 5 and 6 of the previous edition, lays the foundation for later chapters by identifying the key elements of the main approaches to health and sickness.

The inclusion of a new section on the social patterning of health and disease reflects both the centrality of this focus within the sociology of health and illness and the changed political environment following the election of a Labour government in 1997. One of the notable consequences of the latter has been that it is now possible to acknowledge, and begin to address, the profound effects of people's social position in the structure of British society on their health. Chapter 3 examines the relationship between socio-economic status and health in contemporary Britain and discusses the widely used conceptual framework for the recent Acheson Report. Chapter 4 examines the complex relationships between ethnicity and health, focusing primarily upon minority ethnic groups. Chapter 5 looks at the narrowing gap between the health of men and women in our society and the role of changing gender expectations and behaviours upon this. Chapter 6 discusses the relationship between old age and health in contemporary Britain, focusing upon the question of whether increasing life expectancy is necessarily accompanied by longer periods of chronic illness and disability.

Despite the increasing emphasis upon health promotion and prevention and the responsibility of individuals and families for the care of illness, the major part of nursing work continues to be the care of people who are sick. Therefore, the focus of the third section of the book, as in the previous editions, is on the patterns and experience of long-term illness, mental disorder and death and dying. Chapter 7, focusing on chronic illness and physical disability and the ways that these are shaped and given meaning in social interaction, contains new material on the body, self and identity in chronic illness and disability. Chapter 8, examining mental disorders, contains a new and extended discussion of de-institutionalisation and the gap between the principles and practice of care in the community. Chapter 9, considering how and where death and dying are dealt with in contemporary Britain, also reviews important new understandings of bereavement and controversial issues surrounding euthanasia and end-of-life care.

Since the second edition was published in 1997 there have been further changes in the organisation of the NHS that have had profound effects upon those using health services, health care professionals and others caring for the sick. This is reflected in the final section of the book. Chapter 10 provides a background for understanding the social context of health and health care in contemporary Britain, discusses continuing pressures on the NHS and outlines the main elements of the 'mixed economy' of health care. Chapter 11 on health policy adopts an historical perspective to analyse patterns of crisis and reform in the NHS and concludes with an analysis of the Labour government's reforms. The final chapter looks at changes in nursing, paying particular attention to the changing division of labour in nursing and the relationship between medicine and nursing.

Steve Taylor and David Field

List of Contributors

ELLEN ANANNDALE, *BSc, MA, PhD*, Senior Lecturer, Department of Sociology, University of Leicester.

KEN BLAKEMORE, *BA, MSocSci, PhD*, Senior Lecturer, Department of Social Policy, University of Swansea.

DAVID FIELD, *BA, MA, AM, PhD*, Visiting Professor, Department of Epidemiology and Public Health, University of Leicester.

MICHAEL P. KELLY, *BA, MPhil, PhD*, Director of Research and Information, Health and Development Authority and Visiting Professor, London School of Hygiene and Tropical Medicine, University of London.

STEVE TAYLOR, *BA, LLB, MPhil, PhD*, Senior Lecturer, London School of Economics and Coventry University.

Part I
Introduction

Chapter 1
Sociology, Social Research and Health

Sociology originated in western Europe in the nineteenth century at a time of unprecedented social upheaval. Agricultural production was giving way to industrialisation, increasing numbers of people were moving from rural to urban areas and traditional institutions of power, such as the Church and the aristocracy were losing much of their influence. The fact that societies could be transformed so quickly led some people to start asking fundamental questions about the nature of social order and social change and the extent to which people's behaviour is shaped by the societies in which they live. Sociology developed out of these concerns.

This chapter will:

- Introduce readers to sociology and 'sociological problems'
- Explain some fundamental principles and techniques of social research
- Introduce some key theoretical ideas in sociology
- Outline some of the applications of sociology to the study of health, sickness and health care

What is sociology?

There is no clear and simple definition of sociology. The word sociology comes from a combination of the Latin *socius* (meaning companion) and the Greek *logos* (meaning the study of), so the word literally means the study of companionship, or *social relations*. These may be *direct*, face-to face relationships, such as those we have with people in our family or at our college, or they may be *indirect*, as the actions and decisions of people not known to us personally can have an important influence on our life. For example, decisions of health policy makers can bring about significant changes in nurses' working conditions, their professional practice and the nature of their relationships with patients. The fact that social relationships take many different forms means that the scope of sociology is very wide. Thus, the sociology of health and health care can range from things like large scale social and economic developments that affect the health of millions of people, to the study of social organisations, such as hospitals, right down to nurse–patient conversations on a hospital ward. However, the key idea behind sociology is that people's lives and behaviour cannot be divorced from the social contexts in which they participate, directly or indirectly.

Sociologists want to know more about these social contexts. Social relationships are rarely random. Normally they are *organised* in various ways. Family life, education and religious practice are examples of distinct forms of social organisation where behaviour tends to be regular or patterned. For example, you will know from your own experiences that college life tends to follow certain regular patterns. Sometimes this is the result of the *formal organisation* of the college, such as the demands of the syllabus or the times classes start and end. However, a great deal of social organisation is *informal*. For example, in their free time students tend to socialise with the same people in the same places. Sociologists are interested in examining different forms of social organisation, comparing them and explaining the relationships between them. For example, how do changes in economic production, like the introduction of new technologies, or changes in cultural values, affect things like the organisation and delivery of health care?

Sociological problems

It is often thought that sociology is about studying *social problems;* that is things that people feel are going 'wrong' with society, such as increasing crime, poverty, drug abuse and so on. Sociologists are interested in social problems, but sociology is about much more than this. Sociologists are just as interested in things that are generally seen to be 'good', 'right', 'acceptable', 'normal', and 'ordinary'. For example, they examine why people break the 'rules' of a society by committing crimes or behaving in odd, anti-social ways, but they are also interested in the rules themselves and how they work. As the renowned American sociologist Peter Berger (1973) put it:

> 'The fundamental sociological problem is not crime but law, not divorce but marriage, not racial discrimination but racially defined segregation, not revolution but government.'

Sociological problems, then, are about how societies, or parts of societies, work in the way they do. *Thinking sociologically* means being curious about the order of everyday social life, how this order changes and its relationship to the behaviour of individuals.

Social order and social change

Next time you find yourself in a place with lots of people, such as a busy street, a shopping mall or crowded hospital waiting area, just take a few minutes to stop and look. Imagine you are a stranger seeing it all for the first time. You will see evidence of the social order that is all around you. Cars stopping at the red light, people paying for the goods they take from the shops (most of the time!) and patients waiting for their turn to see the doctor or nurse. Most people take this order for granted and the only time they notice it is when someone breaks a rule by driving through a red light, taking goods without paying or going straight to the front of a queue. However, sociologists *begin* by asking questions about the regularity of social life. Why do most people seem to follow the rules of a society or social group most of the time? Where does this order come from? Are these rules generally agreed, or are some groups imposing their rules on others?

Government statistics provide more evidence of the regularities of social life. For example, economic data show that the patterns of employment, production and the exports of a country stay much the same from one year to the next. Demographic data – that is information about the distribution of populations – show that in any given country roughly the same number of people are born each year, get married or get divorced. In health research, the statistics show not only that in any society the numbers of people falling ill, getting better or dying, are much the same year in and year out, they also reveal that there are significant and consistent variations *between* different social groups. For example, those from economically poorer social backgrounds – sometimes referred to in sociology as socially *deprived* or lower *social class* – are more likely to have lower expectations of health, have worse health and, on average, die at a younger age.

Sociology is about identifying and explaining these regularities. So whereas journalists, the mass media and to some extent the general public, are more interested in the *unusual* and the troublesome, sociologists are more interested the usual, the everyday, the taken for granted. However, the social orders sociologists study are constantly changing and sociological research often involves looking back to the past to try to explain these changes. For example, the terms health and illness seem clear enough, but in fact people's views of what constitutes 'health' and 'illness' change over time. Many things that were simply seen as part of everyday life a century ago in Britain, such as pregnancy, long term unhappiness, disruptive behaviour in school and loss of libido in later life, are now seen as medical conditions requiring treatments. Sociologists use the term *medicalisation* to describe the ways in which the scope of medical diagnoses has expanded to include more and more areas of social life. This then raises further questions, such as why aspects of life are being medicalised, how it happens, and what the benefits and drawbacks of medicalisation are. Sociological thinking, then, often involves developing ideas that help explain societies, or parts of them, as continually changing *social processes*.

The individual and society

Commonsense thinking holds that societies are all about individuals. Many social scientists and scientists would agree with this, arguing that as societies are clearly created by individuals, it is the study of the individual – through biology, medicine and psychology for example – that provides the key to understanding human behaviour. In questioning this view sociologists are not, as some claim, rejecting the study of the 'individual' in favour of the 'group'. In fact, sociologists are interested in studying individuals and a great deal of their research involves talking to, and observing, individuals. Sociological research involves seeing the relationship between the individual and wider society as a two-way, rather than a one-way, street. Individuals obviously create societies but sociologists argue that, in important respects, individuals are also shaped by societies in which they live.

As societies evolve, certain ways of behaving become accepted as normal, such as speaking a particular language or people organising themselves into small groups called families. Sociologists use the term *institutionalisation* to describe the processes where certain social practices become accepted ways of doing things in a society or social group (Albrow 1999). These social practices, and the values and beliefs surrounding them, make up the *culture* of a society and these cultural practices and values place expectations on how people should behave. The term *socialisation* describes the various ways people learn about, and generally conform to, these expectations. Socialisation processes begin from the time we are born, but continue in different ways throughout our lives. For example, becoming a student, a nurse or a mother not only involves learning new skills but also behaving in ways that are subject to the social expectations of others.

Sociologists would not, for example, explain the generally negative images of the elderly in modern societies merely in terms of biological decline (see Chapter 6). They would explore social *expectations* surrounding ageing and the elderly. As most elderly people are no longer economically productive, they are usually seen as less valuable. Their care and welfare is also often seen as a 'social problem' and the media, politicians and policy makers sometimes talk of the 'burden', or 'costs', of providing care for the elderly. Once people become 'old' they are usually expected to dress and behave in ways that are seen as appropriate to their status. For example, the elderly are not expected to fall in love, kiss passionately in public places, or wear up-to-date designer clothes. Growing old is not, therefore, *just* a product of biology, it is also a product of social relations. People do not just become old, they also learn to be old by adapting their behaviour to the expectations of others. Thus an *individual's* experiences of growing old will inevitably be influenced by the dominant views that a society holds about ageing.

Sociological problems, then, involve exploring the order and regularity of social life, asking how this order changes over time and examining how individual behaviour is shaped by social relations. However, sociology has to do more than ask interesting questions, it also has to come up with some answers and this involves doing research.

Some principles of social research

In attempting to explain how societies, or parts of societies, work in the way they do, sociologists attempt to go beyond *subjective* opinion, speculation and preference and provide more *objective* accounts of social life. Rather than snatching at pieces of evidence that happen to fit the point they are making, as people tend to do in everyday life, sociological research involves the *systematic* accumulation and interpretation of evidence. This section looks at some of the ways they go about doing this.

Concepts and indicators

If a group of nurses who work together in the same hospital ward were asked to write an account of a particular working day, their accounts would probably be very different. First, they might write about different things, depending on what they felt was important. Secondly, even when they were writing about the same incident, they would probably interpret it differently. People's accounts of things tend to be different because they are selective reconstructions of some set of real events, and the selection process is shaped by people's *subjective* views of what they consider to be important and interesting. Sociologists also have to *select* evidence, but they try to make this selection process more systematic and reliable. One of the ways they try to do this is by using concepts and indicators.

Concepts are clear definitions, or labels, that sociologists give to aspects of the social world that have common features. Social class is an example of a concept in sociology. Social classes are groups of people who share a similar economic position in a society. Many studies have explored the relationship between social class health and health behaviour (see Chapter 3). However, if sociologists want to study this relationship statistically, they have to devise ways of measuring the concepts of class and health in much the same way that the mercury in the thermometer measures the concept of temperature.

These measuring devices are called indicators. As occupation is the major source of income for most people, sociologists have used various forms of 'occupational ranking' as indicators of class, while rates of mortality (death) and morbidity (illness) are commonly used as indicators of health. By looking at average death rates and illness rates in each occupational group, sociologists have been able to examine the relationship between 'class' and 'health' in a systematic way that can then be checked and developed by other researchers.

Comparative methods

The experimental method, which is the basis of scientific research, has limited scope in sociological research. First, it would normally be unethical to conduct experiments on large groups of people without their consent. Secondly, even when experiments are conducted in conditions that resemble the closed world of the laboratory, the results may lack ecological validity as there is no guarantee that people would behave in the same way in the real world.

However, sociologists sometimes interpret data to make comparisons between different populations in ways that resemble the logic of the experiment. For example, in his pioneering study of suicide, Durkheim (1952) discovered that European countries that were predominantly Catholic, such as Italy, had much lower suicide rates than countries that were predominantly Protestant, such as Germany. But was this due to religion or national culture? In order to find out, Durkheim then looked at the suicide rates of Catholic and Protestant regions within countries. The fact that the Catholic rates were still much lower, even with nationality 'controlled', led him to conclude that the relationship between religion and suicide was real rather being an artefact (i.e. the result of some other cause).

Models in sociology

The real social world is never as clear as it is in the concepts and theories of sociologists. However, this is not a criticism of sociology. Even if it was possible, it is not the job of sociology to try to reproduce the complexities of the real social world. Rather, sociologists try to simplify and clarify these complexities. One of the ways they do this is by using theoretical models. A model is a simplified description of some aspects of a society. For example, in attempting to understand and explain social inequality, Marx developed a two-class model of inequality (Crompton 1999). This model held that there was a fundamental division in societies between those who owned the means of generating wealth (ruling class) and those who had only their labour power to offer (subordinate class). Marx was not suggesting that class divisions were really as simple as that in the societies he studied. There were obviously all sorts of 'intermediate strata', such as small traders, professionals and skilled workers. However, in his research he used the two-class model as a starting point to illustrate the extent to which patterns of inequality were shaped by the ownership of the means of economic production.

Reliability and validity

Reliability is about whether the results of the study are repeatable. For example, the concept of social class, described above, can be applied to different societies or to the same society over time. The data would be seen as reliable if different researchers using the concept came up with the same results. For research to be potentially reliable, researchers have to spell out the procedures by which the data was obtained. This is known as *transparency* in social research. Research is valid if the data represents what it is supposed to represent. For example, in his study of suicide, Durkheim used statistics from different countries to test his theory. Other sociologists have criticised this method, arguing that such comparisons are not valid, because the officials in different countries have different procedures for determining whether or not a death is suicide. Durkheim was not, therefore, comparing like with like. The issue of validity illustrates one of the reasons why sociologists are so concerned with method. Data cannot simply be taken at 'face value', researchers also have to find out *how* it was collected in order to assess its validity.

Doing social research

It is important that sociologists do not just present their findings but also explain how they were obtained in order to give others the opportunity to make a more informed judgement of their value. All aspects of social life are of potential interest to sociologists, and data is gathered from a wide range of sources. Sociologists may use *secondary* sources, that is data already in existence, or they may collect their own *primary* data. Another important distinction is between *quantitative* data, that can be measured, and *qualitative* data that cannot be analysed statistically.

Quantitative data

Official statistics

The term official statistics refers to the mass of data collected by the state and other related agencies. For example, a national census is held in Britain every ten years. This provides information about the composition of the population in terms of factors such as births, marriages, divorces, ethnicity and the structure of families. State sources also regularly produce economic statistics on patterns of employment, unemployment, income, expenditure, as well as rates of crime, illness, suicides and the like. In addition to state generated data, other organisations such as hospitals, economic organisations and child protection agencies can be important sources of information for researchers.

Official statistics are widely used by sociologists. They are readily available, comprehensive and allow for trends to monitored over time. A great deal of the information used by many of the studies discussed in this book comes from various forms of official statistics, particularly statistics on patterns of health and illness and their relationship to social factors. However, it is important to remember that just because something is 'official' and expressed in statistical form does not necessarily make it valid and reliable. Statistics are not self-evident 'facts', they are products of the conceptual categories used by the officials who collect them. For example, we may read that working-class people are twice as likely on average to die before middle-class people. However, before we can attach any value to the statistics, we need to know things like what concept of 'class' was being used and what proportions of the population are in these classes. There may also be problems in the collection of some sets of statistics that make their value for research questionable. For example, it is generally accepted in social research that official statistics on things like crime, mental illness and suicide not only underestimate the extent of the problem but may also be systematically biased, as some types of case are much more likely to be reported than others. Therefore, using official statistics in social research not only requires interpreting statistical trends, it also involves understanding *how* the data is produced and evaluating its use for research purposes.

Survey research

One of the most common ways that sociologists generate their own (i.e. primary) data is to ask people questions. In quantitative research this involves using survey methods. In the survey respondents are asked a set of identical questions in exactly the same way and select their responses from a limited range of answers. Surveys can be administered by face-to-face interviews or by asking people to fill in a questionnaire.

Imagine a researcher is using survey methods to examine nurses' views of their working conditions in a particular health authority. While the surveys could be distributed to nurses who happened to be around at the time, it would be difficult to generalise the results as the sample surveyed will almost certainly not be *representative* of the population being studied. To obtain a representative sample the researcher has to use various sampling techniques, such as random sampling where every nurse in the authority has an equal chance of being selected. The more the nurses surveyed reflect the general population of the region, especially in terms of key variables like age, class background, ethnicity, gender, professional status and so on, the more confident the researcher would feel in generalising from the results. The survey is one of the most common tools of social research. It is reliable, transparent, allows large numbers of people to be questioned relatively quickly and cheaply and, because the range of permitted responses is specific and limited, the results can be systematically quantified and analysed.

Survey research also has certain limitations. It lacks flexibility and depth, the questions and range of answers may not reflect the respondents' experiences and it has difficulty accounting for the range of meanings that people give to their actions. To write survey questions and answers the researcher has to use words, but the same word can *mean* different things to different respondents. For example, in a survey of patients' views of their health care, respondents can interpret the word 'satisfied' in many different ways. Sometimes, researchers try to account for this problem of meaning by leaving space for respondents to elaborate their answers. However, because the survey method means that researchers are detached from the people they are studying, it is difficult for them to appreciate how their subjects *really* feel and impossible for them to know how they actually *behave* in real situations. These limitations of the survey, and of quantitative methods in general, mean that some questions have to be examined by alternative, qualitative research strategies.

Qualitative data

Whereas quantitative methods emphasise the *detachment* of researchers, qualitative methods involve researchers *immersing* themselves in the world of their subjects. Imagine a researcher is studying a disabling condition such as rheumatoid arthritis. Quantitative techniques – properly applied – provide important information about things like the prevalence of rheumatoid arthritis in a society, statistical links between the condition and social factors and the resources available for the care and support of sufferers in different areas. However, there are certain questions quantitative techniques cannot answer very well. For example, what is it actually like to have rheumatoid arthritis? How do people experience the condition, negotiate changes in their relationships and come to terms with the restrictions it imposes on their lives? How do they actually behave with their professional and lay carers? Such questions can only be answered by research techniques that bring researchers into much closer contact with those they are studying, such as observing social interaction or interviewing people at great length.

In qualitative research studies sociologists are trying to reproduce aspects of the 'lived experience' of the subjects. The aim is not so much to look for relationships between variables, but to try to understand the viewpoint of those being studied. Rather than use representative samples of larger populations, they are more likely to involve detailed analysis of particular *case studies*. Research reports are usually in the form of a narrative, with the key evidence, such as detailed descriptions of particular episodes or interview extracts, being used to illustrate the point the researcher is making. The validity of qualitative research studies comes from the depth and detail of the researcher's account. Some studies may be further validated by something called respondent validation, where the researcher's interpretations are put back to the group being studied for their comments, criticisms or confirmation.

Observational methods

Observation is a key technique of qualitative research. Observational researchers may be non-participants and simply observe social interaction from a distance, or they may be participant observers who are involved in the actions of those they are studying. This latter technique was first used by western anthropologists who joined tribal societies, learning their language and customs in order to document ways of life that were disappearing with colonisation and the relentless advance of industrialisation. Similarly, in the study of contemporary societies, sociologists have to gain access to the groups or organisations they wish to study and, like the anthropologists, observe and make detailed records of the customs and 'ways of life' of those they are studying.

Although observational studies aim to describe things as they really are, there is the problem that those being observed may change their behaviour because they are being studied. Sometimes researchers try to get round this 'observer effect' by concealing their true identity from the group being studied. For example, in his classic study of a state mental hospital in the United States, Goffman (1991) worked as a games teacher in the institution. However, such 'undercover' research raises ethical issues, as those being studied have not given their consent to the research. In such cases, researchers have to ask themselves whether or not the potential value of the research findings justifies the deception involved (Goode 1996).

There is a richness of detail in observational research that tends to be lacking in other methods. Sociologists are able to see how people behave for themselves rather than relying on official statistics or what they are told in interviews. However, like all methods, observational research has its limitations. Not only is it time-consuming, but the data is hard to test and replicate. Furthermore, there are many areas of social life – domestic violence, sexuality, suicide and childhood experiences for example – that can not usually be studied in this way.

Qualitative interviews

Qualitative researchers also make great use of interviews. However, unlike the formal structured interviews used in survey methods, qualitative interviews are much more like ordinary conversations. There is no set interview structure, no boxes to tick, little input from the researcher and interviewees answer in their own words. The effectiveness of qualitative interviews often depends on the rapport and trust that is built up between researcher and respondent. The aim of such interviews is to allow respondents to reconstruct their experiences in as much detail as possible, giving the researcher, and ultimately the reader, an insight into how *they* experienced particular events. This is illustrated by the following extract from Field (2001) on nursing the dying:

> 'I remember very clearly a patient on geriatrics. I had nursed him on nights and I went back on days – he was double sided CVA. He was very incoherent.... So I just sat with him and held his hand. And I remember the staff nurse coming in asking me if I had nothing better to do. So I said "No. Not at this moment, no." So she said "Would you mind finding something to do?" I really hated her because this man was dying. I'd been with him all this time and why should he die alone?'

While providing much more depth than survey methods, qualitative interviews also have important limitations. Data collection is usually unsystematic and thus hard to generalise from and, as there is far too much data to reproduce, readers are dependent on the *researcher's* selection of data.

Documents

Documents provide a rich source of information for sociologists (Scott 1990). They may include the reports of various government institutions, records from schools, hospitals, law courts and so on, as well as films, photographs, reports from journals, magazines and newspapers. A great deal of historical work, in particular, is based on careful collection and analysis of documentary evidence.

Qualitative researchers may also use personal documents, such as case histories, letters, diaries and autobiographical works that help to tell the 'inside story' of how people have interpreted the situations in which they have found themselves. Documentary evidence can be used to supplement observational or interview data, or be used where neither method is possible. For example, the autobiographical accounts by adults who have tried to harm themselves, been anorexic or been abused in their childhood provide an invaluable source of information for sociologists researching these areas. Similarly, those researching patient care (and health care professionals themselves) can learn a great deal about the experience of being a patient from autobiographical and semi-autobiographical works such as, Solzhenitsyn's *Cancer Ward* or Kesey's *One Flew Over the Cuckoo's Nest.*

Selection of research methods

In comparing different research methods, it is not a question of which method is right or wrong, or better or worse. It is rather that some methods are better suited to some problems than others and this will influence the researcher's selection. For example, a large-scale study of the relationship between the distribution of income and patterns of health and disease will almost certainly use official statistics, whereas a study of how a clinic or hospital ward works will usually involve some form of observational research. Selection of methods is also influenced by external factors, such as whether or not researchers can get direct access to those they want to study, the time and money available, the nature of the audience they are writing

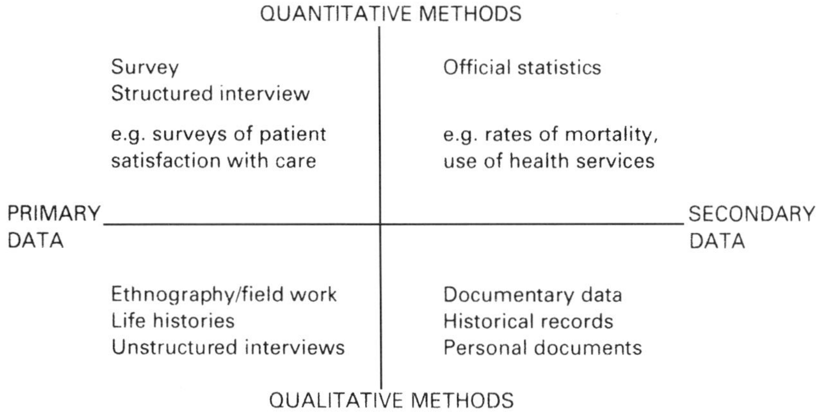

QUANTITATIVE METHODS

Survey Structured interview	Official statistics
e.g. surveys of patient satisfaction with care	e.g. rates of mortality, use of health services

PRIMARY ———————————————————————— SECONDARY
DATA   DATA

Ethnography/field work Life histories Unstructured interviews	Documentary data Historical records Personal documents

QUALITATIVE METHODS

Fig. 1.1   Sources of data in social research.

for and the requirements of those funding the research. The relationship between different sources of data is illustrated in Figure 1.1.

In practice most researchers tend to use a combination of quantitative and qualitative methods. Evidence gained from several different methods usually gives a much fuller and clearer understanding of a subject. The findings from one method can sometimes also be checked with data from another method. For example, researchers could use survey methods to elicit the views of a large number of nurses about their working conditions and then carry out observational case studies of some of the same nurses at work. This will give them a much wider perspective on the research problem. Furthermore, if the things nurses were saying about their work tended to be confirmed by observing nursing practice, then the researchers would be much more confident about the validity and reliability of their findings. However, it is also important to realise that research questions and strategies are not just influenced by practical and methodological issues. They are also shaped by theoretical issues.

Theory in sociology

Theory and method

Doing sociological research is not just about gathering data through various research methods, it is also about developing *theoretical* ideas that describe and explain different aspects of social life. Theory and method are inextricably inter-linked as theoretical ideas guide both the collection and interpretation of data (Marsh 2002).

First, theoretical ideas are needed to *describe* the aspects of society the sociologist is studying. Suppose researchers are studying the relationship between illness and relative poverty. Before any data can be collected they have to use a concept of 'social class', or 'social deprivation', and these are *theoretical* definitions. They then have to identify the indicators they are using to measure the concept. Similarly, they have to define what they mean by 'illness' and how it is to be measured. For example, is the researcher to include all illnesses – in which case things like having a bout of flu and experiencing heart disease would count in the same figure – or just concentrate on 'serious' illnesses? If it is the latter, what is to be counted as 'serious' illness? Once illness has been defined how is it to be measured? Researchers could use a subjective definition and ask people if they have experienced illness, or they could use more objective measures, such as medical records, or periods in hospital. The permutations are endless, but the point is that doing the research involves using *theoretical* notions of 'social class', or 'social deprivation', and 'illness'. Data, then, does not consist of self-evident 'facts' simply waiting to be collected like apples off a tree. It is *constructed* through researchers' theoretical ideas and research strategies. Different theoretical ideas may well produce different 'facts'. This is not to suggest that there is not *really* a relationship between relative poverty and illness, but rather it can *only* be examined systematically through theoretical ideas. All data is therefore theory-dependent.

Secondly, theories are necessary to *explain* why things happen. Suppose the researchers do find reliable and systematic evidence of a relationship between low social class and high levels of illness. This is not an explanation as 'the facts never speak for themselves'. For example, the higher rates of illness amongst the poor can be interpreted in several ways. It may be the result of poor living conditions, inadequate health care, less healthy behaviour amongst the poor, such as higher rates of smoking, or it could be due to genetic influences, with families prone to more illness drifting down to lower socio-economic positions (Chapter 3).

In short, there are usually many different ways in which a piece of evidence can be explained. Part of the researcher's task may be to try to 'adjudicate' between competing explanations by generating further data to show the extent to which different theories fit the available evidence. However, it is important to recognise the limits of sociological explanation as well as its potential. While sociology offers much more than opinion and common sense, it can never achieve the precision and prediction found in the natural sciences, such as physics or biology, as theories cannot be evaluated under controlled experimental conditions. As such sociology offers interpretations of the social world rather than demonstrable universal truths. As Pawson (1999) observes:

'Sociological research will always be partial and provisional and never uniform and universal. I figure that certainty requires humility and that sociological research can only help us in choosing between theories rather than proving one. I rest content that good quality research comes with qualifications – our hypothesis will work only for certain people in certain circumstances at certain times.'

Theoretical divisions in sociology

So far we have been looking at things that are common to sociology. However, it is also important to understand that there is no single sociological approach but rather a number of different theoretical perspectives (Swingewood 1999). Analysis of the different theoretical approaches in sociology cannot be undertaken here, but two of the most important theoretical divisions in sociology concern different views about *what* societies are and *how* to find out about them. In terms of the first question, a broad distinction can be made between sociological theories that define societies as social structures and those that define them as the products of the actions of individuals. In terms of finding out about societies, there is a division in sociology about the extent to which the methods of the natural sciences are applicable in sociology.

Societies as social structures

Some sociological approaches argue that human societies are best understood as social structures, that is as networks of social institutions and patterns of social relationships that are comparatively long lasting. Sociologists adopting this approach attempt to show the ways that various social structures shape the behaviour of the individuals living within them. The focus is thus on large-scale, or macro-, social processes.

Many of those who founded sociology in nineteenth century Europe viewed societies as social structures. For example, Durkheim (1858–1917) saw the morals and values of a society, transmitted from one generation to the next, as external forces that constrain individuals by regulating their behaviour and by binding them to each other through shared membership of institutions like families and religion (Steadman Jones 2001). Sociological approaches that see values and beliefs as the 'core' element of societies are called *idealist* theories. Durkheim's sociology was an attempt to demonstrate that different institutional structures produce differences in individual behaviour, and his famous study of suicide attempted to demonstrate that social groups with more integrating social structures have lower suicide rates.

Marx (1818–93), another founder of sociology, viewed social structures in a rather different way. For him, the key to understanding societies lay in their economic structures rather than their values and beliefs. This is known as a *materialist* approach. Marx claimed that social change was caused by changes in the underlying economic structure of societies rather than by the outcomes of battles or the decisions of powerful people. He argued that the change from agricultural to industrial production brought about a new type of industrial-capitalist society based on the free exchange of goods and services.

Despite the differences between Durkheim's idealist theory focused on cultural values and beliefs and Marx's materialist theory based on economic production, both viewed individual behaviour as the product of the structural organisation of societies. Sociologists studying health and illness from a structural perspective would thus be interested in how things like the culture, class structure or education system of a society influence people's health behaviour, their vulnerability to disease and the organisation of health care.

Societies as products of social action

Social action theory describes theoretical approaches that focus primarily on the meanings and motives behind the actions of individuals. Action theorists argue that as human societies are produced by the intentional activities of people, sociologists should begin by studying individual social action and the meanings behind these actions. Action theorists sometimes accuse structural theorists of reducing people to mere puppets of society. For example, Weber (1864–1920) disagreed with Marx that the rise of industrial capitalist society in western Europe could be explained merely by changes in the economic structure. He argued that this approach did not explain the *motivation* of so many of the early industrial capitalists to work long hours and re-invest, rather than spend, their profits. Weber used statistical and documentary sources to suggest that an important motivating factor in the success of many of the early industrial capitalists was a staunch belief in the Protestant doctrine of predestination, where economic (or worldly) success came to be interpreted as a sign of God's favour. By focusing more on the actions of individuals and the meanings they gave to those actions Weber was able to highlight something that had been absent in Marxism and economic theory, the relationship between religion and the rise of modern capitalism.

Sociologists studying health and illness from a social action perspective are interested in exploring things like how people come to define themselves as healthy or sick, individual experiences of health and illness or day-to-day interactions between health professionals. This kind of research may reveal certain patterns or regularities that might *then* be linked to structural factors, such as family type or social background. Thus it is not that action theorists ignore structure, or structural theorists ignore action, rather it is that they approach the problem of the relationship between the individual and society in different ways.

A science of society?

Many of the earliest sociologists believed that by diligently applying principles that had been so successful in the natural sciences, sociology would be able to discover 'laws' of social order and social change that could then be used to improve societies. Contemporary sociologists are neither so ambitious nor so optimistic. However, many believe that it is still possible to study social life in a relatively objective and scientific way. This involves sociologists maintaining a scientific detachment and describing and explaining regularities of social life in terms that can be measured and tested out by other researchers. Sociologists adopting this view thus have a strong preference for quantitative methods. From this point of view rates of health and disease, for example, are seen as objective realities whose statistical distribution can be correlated with other factors such as social background, housing or type of employment.

Other sociologists are much more sceptical about the application of scientific methods to the study of societies. This approach is sometimes called interpretivist, or subjectivist. Interpretivists emphasise the differences between the study of the natural and social worlds. Unlike the atoms studied by physicists, for example, people engage in conscious intentional activity and, through language, attach meanings to their actions. Thus states of health and illness, for example, are not simply natural phenomena, they are also products of social definition; their meaning is given by social norms and values and these norms vary between different social groups and change over time. They argue that the essentially subjective nature of social life effectively precludes the possibility of a science of society. Sociology is, therefore, about interpreting the different ways that people experience the situations in which they find themselves.

Sociologists studying health and illness from this point of view would be more interested in exploring how certain states came to be defined as healthy or unhealthy and how these social definitions influenced people's experiences of particular conditions. As such, interpretivist sociologists have a strong preference for qualitative research methods that bring them into closer contact with those they are studying. Some of the differences between quantitative and qualitative research strategies are summarised in Table 1.1.

Table 1.1 The differences between quantitative and qualitative approaches.

Quantitative	Qualitative
Focuses on a relatively small number of specific concepts	Attempts to understand the entirety of some phenomenon rather than focus on specific concepts
Begins with preconceived ideas about how the concepts are interrelated	Has a few preconceived ideas and stresses the importance of people's interpretation of events and circumstances, rather than the researcher's interpretation
Uses structured procedures and formal 'instruments' to collect information	Collects information without formal, structured 'instruments'
Collects the information under conditions of control	Does not attempt to control the context of the research but, rather, attempts to capture it in its entirety
Emphasises objectivity in the collection and analysis of information	Attempts to capitalise on the subjective as a means for understanding and interpreting human experiences
Analyses numerical information through statistical procedures	Analyses narrative information in an organised, but intuitive, fashion

Source   D.F. Polit & B.P. Hungler (1991) *Nursing Research: Principles and Methods* (4th edn). Lippincott, Philadelphia. (Reproduced by permission of J.B. Lippincott Company.)

Some sociologists have rather entrenched views about the relative merits of structural and action theories and scientific or interpretative methods. However for most sociologists, and for those such as health professionals looking to apply sociological ideas to practice, it is more useful to view them as complementary, each with their own insights and limitations. For example, a structural approach may have to be employed in exploring something like changes in the provision of health, while a social action approach may be helpful in studying something like nurse–client interactions. Similarly, studying the social factors that appear to make disease and premature death more or less likely lends itself to a quantitative approach, whilst patients' experiences of illness and disability may be usefully understood by using qualitative methods.

Sociology applied to health and health care

The working lives of most health professionals consist of a series of cases presenting a succession of specific problems. Patients, or clients, present with specific
symptoms and health professionals give advice and usually offer some form of
personalised treatment based on their specialist understanding of the human body.
Success is usually judged in terms of improvements in the patient's health or, where
cure is not possible, in their comfort. Sociology provides a different way of looking
at health and illness. Instead of focusing on factors within the human body,
sociology explores the social contexts in which people live and their relationship to
health issues. The other sections of the book examine the *application* of sociological approaches to three main areas.

- The distribution of health and illness in societies
- Illness and disabling conditions
- The organisation and delivery of health care

Part II focuses on research showing the extent to which people's health is
influenced by social and cultural factors. Using research based mainly on structural
theories and quantitative methodologies, it examines the relationship between
health and the 'core' social variables of socio-economic background (Chapter 3),
ethnicity (Chapter 4), gender (Chapter 5) and age (Chapter 6). One of the important
implications of this work for health professionals is that improving the health of
populations involves looking beyond individual cases and personalised health care
to the social contexts that may be producing better health for some and worse
health for others.

Part III looks at sociological analyses of illness. Sociologists have examined the
cultural meanings of illness, the settings of care, and illustrated the various ways that
people's experiences of illness are shaped by cultural values and social interaction. It
examines chronic illness (Chapter 7), mental disorders (Chapter 8) and death, dying
and bereavement (Chapter 9). The implication of this work for health professionals is
that the care of the sick is about more than management of symptoms, it also involves
taking account of the social and psychological aspects of sickness.

Part IV examines the organisation and delivery of health care. Professional–
patient/client interactions take place in various organisational settings that then
influence the nature of those interactions. This involves looking at the changes in
contemporary British society and their influence on the organisation of, and
demand for, health care (Chapter 10), as well as government health policies and
their effects on the delivery of care (Chapter 11) and the specific contexts in which
nursing takes place (Chapter 12).

Summary

Sociology is the study of social relationships. It begins by asking fundamental
questions about the nature of social order, social change and the relationship

between individuals and societies. Sociological research involves systematic collection and interpretation of data from a variety of sources, but the social sciences cannot attain the predictive power of the natural sciences. All methods of data collection in the social sciences have their advantages and their limitations and most research involves using a combination of methods. All social research is collected and interpreted in terms of theoretical ideas and sociologists have different ideas about how the relationship between individuals and societies is best conceived and the extent to which the principles of scientific research are applicable to sociology. Sociological ideas have been applied to the distribution of health and disease, experiences of illness and the organisation of health care.

References

Albrow, M. (1999) *Sociology: the Basics*. Routledge, London.

Berger, P. (1973) *Invitation to Sociology*. Penguin, London.

Crompton, R. (1999) Class and Stratification. In: *Sociology: Issues and Debates* (ed. S. Taylor). Palgrave, Basingstoke.

Durkheim, E. (1952) *Suicide: a study in sociology*. Routledge, London.

Field, D. (2001) 'We Didn't Want Him to Die on His Own' – nurses' accounts of nursing dying patients'. In: *Health and Disease: a reader*, 3rd edn. (eds B. Davey, A. Gray & C. Seale). Open University Press, Buckingham.

Goffman, E. (1991). *Asylums, essays on the social situation of mental patients and other inmates*. Penguin, London.

Goode, E. (1996) The ethics of deception in social research: a case study. *Qualitative Sociology*, **19**, 11–33.

Marsh, I. (ed.) (2002) *Theory and Practice in Sociology*. Prentice Hall, Harlow.

Pawson, R. (1999) Methodology. In: *Sociology: Issues and Debates* (ed. S. Taylor). Palgrave, Basingstoke.

Scott, J. (1990) *A Matter of Record: Documentary Sources in Social Research*. Polity Press, Cambridge.

Steadman Jones, S. (2001) *Durkheim Reconsidered*. Polity, Cambridge.

Swingewood, A. (1999) Sociological Theory. In: *Sociology: Issues and Debates* (ed. S. Taylor). Palgrave, Basingstoke.

Further reading

Introductory sociology texts

Haralambos, M. & Holborn, M. (2001) *Sociology: Themes and Debates*, 5th edn. Harper Collins, London.

Taylor, S. (ed.) (1999) *Sociology: Issues and Debates*. Palgrave, Basingstoke.

Research methods

Bryman, A. (2001) *Social Research Methods*. Oxford University Press, Oxford.

Denscombe, M. (2003) *The Good Research Guide*, 2nd edn. Open University Press, Buckingham.

Silverman, D. (2000) *Doing Qualitative Research*. Sage, London.

Health and nursing research

Cormack, D. (ed.) (2000) *The Research Process in Nursing*. Blackwell Science, Oxford.

Roper, J. & Shapira, J. (2000) *Ethnography in Nursing Research*. Sage, London.

Chapter 2
Approaches to Health, Illness and Health Care

For many people the idea of health care still probably conjures up images of doctors and nurses working in surgeries and hospitals, with increasingly complex technology. This is hardly surprising, as the major function of health care systems in modern societies is to try to restore people to health through treatments of one sort or another. However, the activities of health care professionals now go well beyond treating the sick. An increasing number of doctors and nurses are focusing on the 'well' rather than the 'sick'. Screening programmes set out to discover signs of disease before they are presented in the surgery, and people are bombarded with information about what they could, and should, be doing to lead healthier lives. To many observers, this represents a fundamental shift in the way in which contemporary societies approach health and illness.

This chapter will:

- Explain what is meant by a bio-medical model of health
- Discuss socio-medical models of health and their implications
- Introduce the idea that illness is a distinct social role
- Look at the social aspects of the nurse–patient relationship

The bio-medical model of health

The development of medicine is usually described in terms of a series of spectacular breakthroughs, such as Pasteur's development of vaccinations, Fleming's discovery of penicillin or the first heart transplant by Christian Barnard. In this 'heroic' view of medicine, the struggle for better health is seen as a 'war' waged by doctors and medical scientists against an impersonal enemy called disease on the battleground of the human body. The idea that people's health, at least in a relatively affluent society like Britain, is predominantly a reflection of science's understanding of the body, the disease process and the development and availability of effective treatments reflects *a bio-medical model* of health. In this model:

- Health is the absence of biological abnormality
- Diseases have specific causes
- The human body is likened to a machine to be restored to health through personalised treatments that arrest, or reverse, the disease process

- The health of a society is seen as largely dependent on the state of medical knowledge and the availability of medical resources

The bio-medical model of health still underpins the organisation and delivery of health care in contemporary societies. Medical research is focused primarily on bio-chemical or genetic processes underlying disease. Most medical work involves diagnosing and treating abnormalities within the body and hospital-based, high-technology medicine still receives the major share of health care budgets. The education and training of most health professionals – particularly doctors – revolves around understanding the human body and intervening in the disease process, and the most prestigious and highly paid members of the health care professions are the experts in curative medicine, the hospital consultants, and the leaders of medical research teams.

Bio-medical dominance over health and healing was consolidated in the nine-teenth and early twentieth century with the movement of medicine from the bedside to the hospital and the laboratory (Seale *et al.* 2001). During this period there were great advances in medical science, such as the discovery and treatment of bacterial infections, new and safer surgical techniques and developments in pharmacology. It was generally assumed that these advances in clinical medicine played a significant part in the great improvement in health standards that occurred around the same time. This led to the expectation that it was only a matter of time before scientific medicine overcame the diseases of modern society, such as cancer, heart disease, arthritis and mental illness. It was widely anticipated in industrial societies around the middle of the twentieth century that much greater investment in medical research and health care would produce further dramatic improvements in levels of health. But how realistic was this expectation and how valid was the assertion about the past on which it was based? In advanced industrial societies, such as Britain, life expectancy has increased dramatically, but how much of this has been due to clinical intervention and treatment? This question is considered in the following section.

Infectious diseases: the role of medicine

Epidemiology is the study of the distribution of health and disease in populations by using a range of 'health indicators', such as rates of mortality (the proportion of people dying each year). In terms of this criterion Britain, like the rest of the western world, has become much 'healthier' over the past 150 years. In 1851 the annual death rate was 22.7 per 1000 and average life expectancy at birth was around 40 years. By 1950 average life expectancy had increased to over 60 and in the early twenty-first century it is around 80 years (Fig. 2.1).

The dramatic decline in the death rate from the middle of the nineteenth century to the middle of the twentieth century was mainly due to the decline in deaths from infectious diseases (Table 2.1). It was widely believed that clinical measures, in the form of therapy and later immunisation, played a major part in this decline. How-ever, this view was challenged by McKeown (1979). By tracing the history of specific infectious diseases, he was able to show that most of them were declining well *before* effective medical treatment was available (Fig. 2.2). The only exceptions

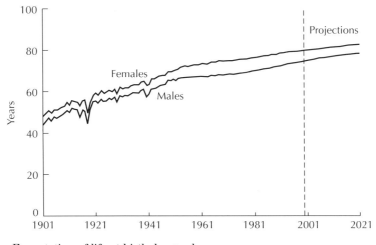

Fig. 2.1 Expectation of life at birth: by gender.
Source *Social Trends* (2002) Crown copyright.

Table 2.1 Reduction of mortality 1848–54 to 1971: England and Wales.

	Percentage of reduction
Conditions attributable to micro-organisms	
(1) Airborne diseases	40
(2) Water- and food-borne diseases	21
(3) Other conditions	13
Total	74
	26
Conditions not attributable to micro-organisms	
All diseases	100

Source T. McKeown (1979) *The Role of Medicine*. Blackwell Publishers, Oxford. (Reproduced by permission of Blackwell Publishers and the University Press of Princeton.)

to this general pattern were smallpox, diphtheria and polio, where immunisation was an important factor. Programmes of immunisation against infection are obviously an important safeguard against the spread of infections, but the fact that clinical intervention seemed to play only a relatively small part in the decline of most infectious diseases suggested that there must be other explanations.

Important public health reforms implemented in the nineteenth century, particularly those leading to cleaner water supplies, were the main reason in reducing exposure to water and food-borne infections such as cholera and typhoid. However, these reforms do not explain the decline in deaths from air-borne infections, such as tuberculosis, that accounted for 40% of the total decline (Table 2.1). According to McKeown, the major reason for the declining death rate was that people became stronger, and thus more resistant to infectious disease, due to better nutrition, improvements in public health and changes in their behaviour, especially greater use of contraception and improved personal hygiene. The limited part played by clinical intervention in the decline of the infectious disease was not unique to

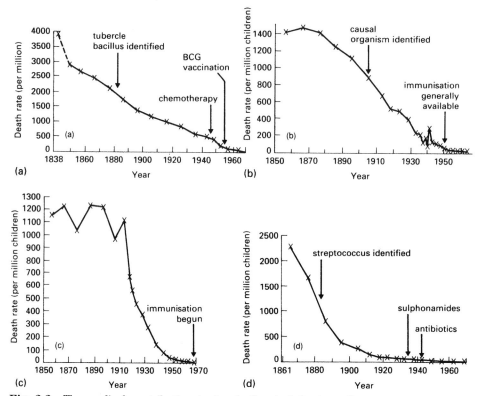

Fig. 2.2 The medical contribution to the decline in infectious diseases. (a) Respiratory tuberculosis: death rates, England and Wales. (b) Whooping cough: death rates of children under 15, England and Wales. (c) Measles: death rates of children under 15, England and Wales. (d) Scarlet fever: death rates of children under 15, England and Wales.
Source McKeown, T. (1976) *The Modern Rise of Population.* Arnold, London. © Thomas McKeown (reproduced by permission of Hodder Arnold).

Britain. For example, McKinlay and McKinlay (1977) came to broadly similar conclusions about the contribution of medicine to improvements in health in the United States. McKeown used his research to criticise the organisation of health care in modern societies. He suggested that modern medicine's preoccupation with the treatment of established diseases was a misuse of health care resources and that the best prospects for improving health in modern societies lay with trying to prevent, or reduce, environmental causes of disease.

McKeown's analysis has been subjected to a number of criticisms. Szreter (1988), reinterpreting the data, has argued that McKeown underestimated the role of medicine in bringing about the public health reforms that, amongst other things, improved the standard of nutrition that helped make people more resistant to disease. It has also been observed that McKeown ignored the fact that thousands of TB patients were incarcerated in institutions, thus limiting the spread the infection and contributing to the declining death rate (Le Fanu 1999). Critics have also argued that by basing his analysis on mortality rates, McKeown failed to take into account the contribution of clinical medicine to improving the *quality* of people's lives by, for example, controlling pain, improving eyesight and restoring mobility. Bunker (2001) goes further, suggesting that many new developments in clinical medicine since McKeown's research in the 1970s have made a significant contribution to longevity as well as quality of life. He cites evidence suggesting that almost 20% of the increase in longevity in the United States and Britain in the twentieth century can be directly attributable to clinical measures. However, despite these reservations, McKeown's research did demonstrate beyond reasonable doubt that health in the past was influenced more by environmental changes than by developments in treatment.

Medicalisation and iatrogenesis

While McKeown was suggesting that clinical medicine has an important but limited part to play in improving health, other critics went much further, arguing that modern medicine's preoccupation with technology and drug therapy has led to an 'epidemic' of *iatrogenic* (i.e. medically caused) disease. Medical accidents, infections acquired in hospital, adverse reactions to drugs and complications following surgery are all examples of iatrogenic disease. For example, it has been estimated that over 10% of hospital patients contracted some form of infection, while a report into peri-operative deaths suggested that the surgical intervention itself was a factor in 30% of deaths and the major factor in 7% of cases (Baggot 1994).

Illich (1990), in a radical critique of modern medicine, extended the concept of iatrogenesis by arguing that the detrimental effects of medicine go beyond direct clinical harm. He accused the 'medical establishment' – by which he meant health care professionals, health administrators, pharmaceutical companies and the suppliers of medical equipment – of creating *social iatrogenesis*, i.e. sponsoring sickness by creating unrealistic health demands that can then only be met by more health care and greater consumption of medical products. Not only are more and more treatments being found for long-established diseases, but more and more aspects of life are also becoming subject to the scrutiny and control of health professionals. Experiences once seen as a normal part of the human condition, such as pregnancy and childbirth, childhood, long-standing unhappiness, ageing and dying have now been brought under medical jurisdiction. Illich claims that these processes of medicalisation are producing a *cultural iatrogenesis* where people 'unlearn the acceptance of suffering as an inevitable part of their conscious coping with reality and learn to interpret every ache as an indicator of their need for padding and pampering'. Illich argued that people should fight back against medical dominance over their lives. Medicine's monopolistic control over health and healing should be abolished, leaving people freer to take more responsibility for their health and health care and, ultimately, for their own lives.

It is important to put the critique of medicalisation into context. First, not only have rates of medical cure increased spectacularly in some areas, such as heart disease, skin cancer and leukaemia but, as we have already observed, many medical treatments contribute a great deal to improving the quality of people's lives. Second, it has been argued that the extent of medicalisation has been exaggerated, and people's capacity to resist medical control underestimated (Williams & Calnan 1996). Finally, even if the medicalisation thesis is accepted – as it is by most sociologists – the increasing consumption of medicines and treatments cannot simply be explained in terms of the 'imperialism' of the 'medical establishment'. This does not explain why so many people in contemporary societies actively seek out and even demand medical solutions to the management of their daily lives.

Some insight into this question may be gained from developing the ideas of one of the founders of sociology, Durkheim. He argued that the process of industrialisation tends to be accompanied by a decline in the influence of social institutions, such as the family, community, and organised religion, that tend to 'bind' people together and give them a common sense of identity and purpose. While this has resulted in greater individual choice and freedom, in times of personal difficulty and crisis increasing numbers of people had fewer sources of help and social support within their immediate environment. From this perspective, the tendency of more people to seek professional help and medication in coping with their lives is not a *consequence* of medicalisation, as Illich argued, but rather a *cause* of medicalisation that has its origins in the changing fabric of modern societies.

Socio-medical models of health

Bio-medicine and the health care practices arising from it occupy a paradoxical position in contemporary societies. On the one hand, there is continued enthusiasm for new medical breakthroughs as people seek treatment for an increasing range of conditions. On the other hand, there is also some disillusionment with clinical medicine and growing distrust of doctors and nurses (Chapter 10). Despite massively increased investments in medical research and health care, most of the diseases of modern society remain stubbornly resistant to effective treatment, let alone cure. As the resources for researching and treating disease become squeezed, the attention of governments and an increasing number of health professionals has turned to the social and environmental influences on health giving rise to a new socio-medical approach to health based on disease prevention and health promotion. In the socio-medical model:

- Health is more than the absence of disease, it is a resource for everyday living
- Diseases are caused by a combination of factors, many of them environmental
- The focus of inquiry is on the *relationship* between the body and its environment
- Significant improvements in health are most likely to come from changes in people's behaviour and in the conditions under which they live

Three inter-related approaches can be distinguished in the socio-medical model. The first focuses on individual behaviour and lifestyle choices. The second explores people's immediate social environment, particularly their relationships with others. The third is more concerned with general socio-economic and environmental influences.

Behavioural approaches

An argument that has become increasingly influential in recent years is that health depends less on what doctors and nurses do for patients and more on what people do for themselves. There is now a mass of evidence linking many of the diseases of modern society to 'behavioural factors', such as sedentary lifestyles, poor diet and widespread use of drugs such as alcohol and tobacco. Smoking, for example, is estimated to contribute to 100 000 deaths a year, while alcohol abuse accounts for a further 10 000. Many doctors and nurses have been at the forefront of campaigns to educate people about the risks of 'unhealthy' behaviour. In this context it has been argued that health professionals are taking over some of the social control functions previously associated with organised religion (Turner 1995). The religious distinction between good and evil is being replaced by the medical distinction between healthy and unhealthy. Whereas religious institutions once warned of the punishments waiting in the afterlife for sinful behaviour, health professionals now warn people of the dangers waiting in this life for unhealthy behaviour. For example, a report by the Royal College of Physicians (1978) into premature deaths concluded:

'Our initial findings will come as no surprise to the profession. Doctors have been saying for years that the causes of many of the diseases of middle life are not mysteries, but are contributed to by overeating, excess alcohol and tobacco.'

On the other hand, good, or healthy behaviour has it rewards. McKeown (1979) cited research that assessed the effects on health of following seven rules:

- Don't smoke cigarettes
- Sleep for seven hours
- Eat breakfast
- Keep weight down
- Drink moderately
- Exercise daily
- Don't eat between meals

The researchers concluded that health and longevity increased with the number of rules followed. Life expectancy at age 45 was 11 years longer for people following six or seven of the rules than for those following less than four. 'Virtue', McKeown observed, 'is not so often so handsomely rewarded'.

The 'health targets' set by the government's *The Health of the Nation* (1992) also followed an essentially behavioural approach. Whilst stating in principle that better health requires a combination of governmental and individual responsibility, in practice the report placed most emphasis on lifestyle factors. For example, the main 'strategies' for combating heart disease and stroke, which together accounted for 38% of deaths in England, were 'to encourage people to stop smoking, increase physical activity and reduce consumption of saturated fatty acids, sodium and alcohol'.

The Health of the Nation also recognised a special role for nurses in health education and health promotion and recent reforms in nurse education and practice put more emphasis on health education. Primary health education is concerned with encouraging people to behave in ways that will help them avoid disease or injury. This involves nurses not only helping to educate individual patients, but also working in schools, colleges and other community institutions developing programmes of education on things such as diet and misuse of drugs. Secondary health education aims to halt or reverse the development of a disease or a condition. This may include the nurse encouraging high-risk groups to make use of screening services, or spotting signs of disability or developmental delay in children. In tertiary health education nurses try to prevent further complications where disease already exists, such as giving guidance about diet to diabetics or helping people adjust to irreversible disability.

Sociologists, while not disputing the influence of behavioural factors on health, have questioned the value of many health education programmes. From a sociological point of view all human behaviour, including health-related behaviour, has to be understood in terms of the social contexts from which it emerges. When studied from the point of view of the people concerned, behaviour that may appear to be 'irrational' from a distance may have a rationality of its own when studied more closely. Smoking behaviour amongst working-class women provides a good example of this.

For many years smoking has been identified as the major preventable cause of death in the developed world. In general people from the working classes have been less responsive to anti-smoking campaigns than people from the middle and upper classes. Working-class women with children have become a priority for health educationalists not only for the harm they may be doing to their own health but also because their children are affected directly by passive smoking and indirectly by socialisation into smoking. From research into women in low income families who were caring for pre-school children, Graham (1994) argued that smoking has to be set in the context of both poverty and motherhood. The mothers who smoked in Graham's study exhibited more stress symptoms than those who did not and smoking was part of a 'strategy' by which they were able to maintain their caring role when their calm broke down. For some women in the study smoking was associated with breaks in caring. As one woman put it, 'I smoke when I'm sitting down, having a cup of coffee, it's part and parcel of resting.' Graham argued that smoking rather than being purely negative, has a paradoxical place in the lives of many of the women she studied. While it clearly increases the risks of ill health, it also helps women cope with caring and, as such, promotes family welfare.

This type of research suggests that behavioural factors cannot easily be separated from the material circumstances of people's everyday existence. Without such understanding it is all too easy to blame people for unhealthy behaviour that may have deeper roots than their fecklessness or ignorance. Health education is clearly very important as the information and guidance it provides can give people more autonomy to make informed decisions about their health. However, a sociological perspective suggests that health education programmes, or the efforts of individual primary health care workers such as community nurses, are more likely to be effective if they place the behaviour into context and take into account the *meaning* that it has for the individuals concerned.

Social relationships and social support

Stress has been described as the epidemic of modern societies. Since the 1960s a number of studies have shown that exposure to stressful life events, such as bereavement, divorce, unemployment or occupational change, financial problems or migration, can make people more vulnerable to disease and even premature death. Researchers are still not entirely sure how people's life experiences influence their physical health, but there is now increasing evidence from the biological sciences suggesting that prolonged exposure to stressful life events produces bio-chemical changes in the body that weaken its immune system and leave the individual more vulnerable to disease. However, while stressful life events are associated with a higher *risk* of disease, they do not *necessarily* cause it and there has been a great deal of research, particularly in biology and psychology, into factors that influence people's ability to adapt to stress. In this context, sociological work has explored the relationship between people's health and their interactive social networks.

More than a century ago, Durkheim (1952) showed that even such an apparently 'individual' act as suicide could be explained sociologically. His research showed that the more people are integrated into the social groups around them – that is, the more their lives are woven into those of others through, for example, kinship bonds or shared membership of organisations – the less vulnerable they are to suicide. In the last three decades sociologists have also demonstrated links between social integration and mental and physical health. In a major longitudinal study in the United States, Berkman and Syme (1979) followed a group of 5000 adults over nine years. They operationalised the concept of integration by using four indicators (see Chapter 1): marriage, regular contact with friends and relatives, church member-ship and membership of voluntary organisations. They then calculated a social network score for each person. After controlling for health status and health behaviour, such as smoking, they found that morbidity and mortality rates for the poorly integrated were between two and three times higher than for those who had high levels of integration. Whilst some researchers have argued that social support provided by integration is of general benefit in promoting health, others have sug-gested that its major benefit is as a 'buffer' in helping people cope with stressful life experiences.

Social support operates at different levels. *Emotional support* can reassure individuals that they are still cared for and give them the opportunity to vent worries and negative feelings. *Instrumental support*, such as physical care, financial assistance or help with responsibilities like child care or shopping, is often essential in helping people get through day-to-day living after a stressful experience. Emo-tional and, to a lesser extent, instrumental support also have the effect of showing people that they are still valued and worthy of the concern of others, and thus help maintain, or re-establish, their sense of self-esteem. Finally, as stressful life events often place people in situations that are unfamiliar to them, *informational support* can be crucial. For example, if a person has become ill, information about diet and medication is often vital to successful adaptation, coping and recovery.

It is perhaps ironic that so many people in contemporary societies seem to be turning their backs on traditional sources of social support when sociologists are discovering just how important they are for health. Nurses and other health workers cannot change societies but they have to try and mitigate the consequences as best they can. One way of doing this is to develop health promotion initiatives that

improve social support networks, especially for the clients or patients from vulnerable and marginalised social groups, such as the elderly, certain ethnic minorities, lone mothers and groups with particular social and psychological problems.
For example, a study of homeless women, many of whom were also drug users,
found that those who had social support from non-users reported better psychosocial profiles and were much more likely to be receptive to drug treatment programmes than those with little or no support (Nyamathi *et al.* 2000).

Social support also appears to be a significant factor in recovery from illness. A
number of studies have shown the importance of social support in helping people
adapt to and make better recoveries from a range of diseases, including various
cancers, heart disease, stroke and depression (Ell 1996). In hospital care the
emotional, instrumental and informational support traditionally given to patients by
nurses is not simply to 'service' biomedical treatment, but is itself a crucial part of
the healing process and should be valued as such. In the community care of people
with long-term illnesses and disabilities, attention is increasingly turning to the
social support networks surrounding the patient.

Most support for people with chronic illnesses or disabilities is provided by
families, and this can place a great deal of strain on the family, particularly the main
caregiver. Social support has two aspects: it is a potential source of health for those
receiving it and a potential source of stress for those providing it. In addition to the
burden of caring, family members may also be confronted by financial strain,
reduced opportunities for recreation and social isolation. The main caregiver, in
particular, may experience depression, a lack of opportunity to express their distress, inadequate support from other family members and a lack of information from
other health professionals, all of which may undermine their continued ability to
provide effective support for the patient.

In the management of long-term illness and disability, support from health professionals for carers can be as important as support for the patient. A number of
studies have shown that social support can mitigate some of the stresses of caring
(Hansell *et al.* 1998). Nurses, in particular, are well placed to provide emotional
support by encouraging carers, listening to their problems and allowing them to
express their feelings about the patient's condition. This may also result in more
open communication between caregivers and patients. Informational support may
focus on discussing the nature of the illness with family members and helping to
plan strategies for some of the problems most likely to be encountered. By identifying the specific help that can most effectively be provided and the progress that
can be realistically expected, nurses may help carers avoid feeling overwhelmed by
the extent of their responsibilities and demoralised by the patient's lack of progress.
Instrumental support for the family may involve, for example, helping to obtain
financial or domestic support, arranging respite care or helping to make contacts
with support groups.

Socio-environmental approaches

While helping people to change their behaviour and support networks can have
obvious benefits for their health, such individualistic approaches have been criti-

cised. First, critics argue that behaviourist approaches overlook the extent to which people's health is linked to factors that are outside their direct control, such as poor housing, hazards at work and environmental pollution. Secondly, attempts to encourage better health behaviour are confronted by a multi-million dollar corporate 'disease promotion' industry, that uses seductive images to persuade people of the pleasure of things like smoking, fast food, alcohol and fast cars. It is argued that rather than 'blaming' individuals, more health promotion action should be directed at restricting access to 'unhealthy' substances and activities by curtailing the activities of the disease promotion industry through government legislation.

Socio-environmental approaches to health are aimed at creating social and environmental conditions that are more conducive to health and the focus is on the social responsibilities of governments and other organisations rather than the responsibilities of individual citizens. This involves joint action from communities, government, voluntary agencies and the health service to create 'healthy alliances'. Socio-environmental health initiatives operate at many different levels. For example, there is now a mass of evidence linking health status to socio-economic position (Graham 2000). In simple terms, people living in the poorer sections of society are more at risk of illness and tend to die younger. In this context, health promotion work involves identifying the causes of these health inequalities, developing policies and strategies to try to reduce them and incorporating them into the education and practice of health professionals. Another set of strategies involves producing healthier environments that maximise the possibilities of leading healthier lives for all citizens. Examples of this are legislation banning smoking from the workplace and many other public areas, measures to reduce traffic speed, especially in built-up areas, and stricter monitoring of industrial waste.

As well as developing national strategies, many health promotion campaigns are targeted at specific social groups or communities, such as a workforce, a minority group, or people living in a particular area. The aim is to help a community, or social group, increase its control over environmental conditions that may be affecting their health. For example, the health education provided by nurses can go beyond informing people of the implications of their own behaviour and include information about the social or organisation factors that may be undermining their health. It could also involve targeting people who have the power to bring about change in an area, such as employers, local government representatives or people in the media. In this respect health workers are encouraged to use a wider definition of health care that incorporates social and political influences on health. This might involve protest action, setting up self-help groups, or arranging meetings with the representatives of the council or health services.

There is clearly great scope for improving health by reforming social and environmental conditions. However, socio-environmental approaches are also open to criticism. First, there is rather more rhetoric than reality. While the literature contains endless definitions of health and health promotion and grandiose ideals of social change, empowerment and partnerships, concrete and testable strategies for health professionals to follow in their day-to-day work are much harder to find. Second, in their desire to distinguish themselves from individualistic behavioural approaches, socio-environmental writers appear to see solutions to health problems solely in terms of political and environmental factors and thus tend to depict people as rather passive victims of 'unhealthy' social arrangements (Kelly 1996). Sociological analysis suggests that such an approach neglects the complexity of the relationship between the individual and society (Chapter 1). People do not simply react to social structures, they are also active agents in their creation and make choices about their behaviour. Third, while behaviourist approaches are based on the idea of individual choice and responsibility, socio-environmental health promotion advocates are more likely to view the state as responsible for the nation's health. Their aim is to convince governments that more unhealthy activities should be either banned or put out of people's reach by price increases. Some critics have argued that such authoritarian measures are incompatible with the guiding principles of a democratic society where people should be free to decide for themselves (Anderson 1991).

Surveillance and social control

The growth of preventative and promotional health care has resulted in increasing numbers of health professionals monitoring apparently healthy people for evidence of risk factors in their bodies, their behaviour or in their social environments. This has been described as *surveillance medicine* (Armstrong 1995). The shift in focus from 'sickness' to 'health' has some important implications for health professionals and for nurses in particular.

First, surveillance medicine gives rise to ethical problems, as nurses become more involved in managing people's lives rather than just their illnesses. For example, many community nurses advise and support families, especially where there are young children. The relationship is based on trust and consent. However, community nurses are also expected to engage in surveillance of families, not only for clear-cut evidence of harm to a child but also for any signs of risk that *may* compromise a child's future safety and welfare. They are then expected to pass on their concerns to multi-disciplinary teams that may include representatives of social services, NSPCC and the police. This potential violation of families' rights – for example the consent they give is not an informed consent – is legitimised by the fact that child care has become medicalised and certain forms of parenting are seen as early symptoms of disease. In this context, Taylor and Tilley (1989) have argued that the surveillance of families without their knowledge or consent not only raises important ethical issues for community nurses, but also threatens the basis of trust on which much of their general work rests.

Secondly, some critics have become concerned about what they see as a tyranny of health promotion where, often on the flimsiest evidence, more and more health hazards are being identified in everyday life (Le Fanu 1999). They argue that health promotion activists create 'health panics' that cause unnecessary worry and make people scared of daily life. This institutionalised paranoia is captured by Reinharz (2001):

'I would like to get through a day without being assaulted by warnings. I find this barrage of dire information intrusive, pervasive and depressing ... the signs, newspaper articles, radio reports and labels tell me to watch out. They let me know that life is dangerous. It's almost foolhardy to be in the sun, to be in a car, or to take food (poison?) from a supermarket shelf. Do I buy margarine or butter knowing, as I have learned, that both are bad?'

It would be ironic if health promotion professionals, in their reaction against the bio-medical model and its limitations, succeed in transforming life itself into a disease.

Thirdly, the key idea behind surveillance medicine is that prevention is better than cure. This is a sensible attitude, but it can also be misleading. While some diseases are clearly preventable, disease and disability, like death, can never be prevented only postponed. Everyone who lives long enough is going to become ill at some time and the majority of health professionals, including the majority of nurses, are going to be involved in one way or another in the treatment and care of the sick. It is thus very important that in its enthusiasm for 'health nursing' rather than 'sick nursing' (Macleod Clark 1993), nurse education does not follow the bio-medical model in overlooking the care of the long-term sick and disabled.

Social aspects of sickness

As societies modernise the burden of disease shifts from acute to chronic (long-term) illness and disability (Chapter 7). While clinical medicine can treat many of these chronic conditions, it cannot cure many of them, and thus more and more people are spending a greater proportion of their lives coping with illness.

Health professionals, and doctors in particular, have been criticised for having a detached, impersonal approach, with the bio-medical model objectifying illness and reducing patients to little more than a collection of symptoms. Critics have argued that more attention should be given to the social, psychological and, more recently, political aspects of illness and disability (Oliver 1996). Both medical and nurse education have begun to respond to this by looking beyond the medical model and adopting a more person-centred approach to patient care. In this context, sociologists are interested in the ways that individual experiences of illness are shaped by wider social contexts, emphasising that the transition from health to illness involves significant changes in social status.

The sick role

Parsons (1951) was one of the first sociologists to conceptualise sickness as a social state. He saw sickness as a potential threat to social order as people were not complying with the work-orientated norms of modern societies. Allocating people to a distinct sick role helped manage this challenge to social and moral order. In Parsons' model the sick role consists of privileges and obligations. Sick people are:

- Exempted from their everyday responsibilities
- Not held responsible for their sickness

- Expected to define sickness as undesirable and be motivated to get better
- Expected to seek professional help and comply with medical advice

Failure to comply with the obligations may result in a loss of the privileges. Parsons also identified a corresponding medical role of privileges and obligations. Doctors have intimate access to patients who therefore have to be protected by doctors':

- Formal education and training
- Objectivity and detachment
- Professional standards and collegiate control
- Ethical obligations to act in the patients' best interests

Although Parsons developed his analysis in terms of doctor–patient relations, it can also be used to help make sense of nurse–patient relations. Nurses have less power than doctors but most of them also work with people who have entered the sick role and, like doctors, they have privileged and often intimate access to patients. Nurse training, the definition of their work as 'patient centred' and their rules of professional conduct also function to regulate professional relations and protect patients from exploitation.

The concept of the sick role has been subjected to a number of criticisms. First, it has been argued that Parsons' model cannot be applied to many chronic illnesses from which patients cannot recover. However, as Parsons observed in a later re-evaluation of the sick role, many people with chronic illnesses are still expected to follow medical advice to control symptoms in a way that mirrors recovery from acute illness. Second, and more significantly, it has been shown that access to the sick role is rather more problematic than Parsons' model assumes. Studies of *illness behaviour*, that is the processes by which people come to define themselves as ill, have shown that only a minority of symptoms, including some quite serious ones, are brought to medical attention. For example, in their classic study of South London, Wadsworth *et al.* (1971) found that although 91% of their sample reported having symptoms of illness, just over a quarter of them were taking no action, over half were self-medicating and only a fifth were having medical treatment. There is thus a distinction between patient's *subjective* experiences of illness and being *objectively* defined by doctors as having a disease. Therefore, it has been suggested that what Parsons is really talking about is *a patient role* rather than a sick role (Turner 1995). Third, in a very influential paper, Szasz and Hollander (1956) criticised Parsons for not analysing the range of possible doctor–patient relationships, and for not recognising that doctors and patients may be more or less active in controlling the encounter. Parsons has also been criticised for assuming an unduly consensual model of the doctor–patient relationship. He showed that there are differences between the knowledge, interests and expectations of doctors and their patients that may lead to tension and conflict. This is equally true for nurse–patient/client relationships, with the additional complication that these are also influenced by relationships between nurses and doctors that have their own tensions and conflicts (Chapter 12).

Despite these valid criticisms of Parsons' formulation of the sick role, it is still seen as a major contribution to the sociology of health and illness. First, it helps to explain differential access to health care and also how certain categories of patients are treated differently by health care staff. For example, in a study of a casualty department, Jeffrey (2001) found staff referring to some patients, such as those who had been hurt while drunk and the repeated overdosers, as the 'rubbish'. What characterised the 'rubbish' was that, like the heavy and unrepentant smokers who are pushed to the back of waiting lists for cardiac surgery, they were seen to have been largely responsible for their own condition and therefore not legitimately sick. Secondly, whereas the bio-medical model focuses exclusively on the sick person, and their body in particular, Parsons' recognition that sickness is a social state with distinct cultural expectations draws attention to *the role of others* in the process of becoming ill. From this perspective, sociologists are interested in exploring social reactions to sickness and disability and how these reactions shape people's experiences of illness and, ultimately, of themselves.

Social reactions to sickness

Sickness labels can easily become what sociologists call a dominant status; that is, the illness or disability comes to be seen by others – and sometimes by the person themselves – as a major source of their identity. Even if the person has a high profile in some other area, they may still be seen as a disabled actor or a diabetic footballer for example. As illness labels are typically seen as such a powerful statement of a person's identity, there is an understandable tendency – even amongst health care professionals – to view a person's, or patient's, behaviour in terms of their condition. For example, an outburst of anger by a person with severe physical disabilities may well be rationalised by staff as an understandable consequence of the frustration of being disabled, even though the anger may be caused by something else. It is therefore important for health professionals to try to distinguish between the *person* and the *condition* rather than assuming that one is simply a consequence of the other.

Sickness and disabling conditions are often *stigmatising*. People are socially stigmatised when they are seen by others to be in some way unacceptable or inferior and are thus denied full social acceptance (Goffman 1990). In stigma there is a discrepancy between what Goffman calls a person's 'virtual social identity' (the way they should be if they were normal) and their 'actual social identity' (the way they are). Those who are stigmatised are confronted with a series of decisions about their 'spoiled identity' both in terms of their interactions with others and their own self-concept. People are more likely to experience stigmatised reaction from others when their impairment is visible. In Goffman's terms, they are 'discredited' and this may lead to withdrawal from social participation, especially in public areas. When the condition is not visible, as in epilepsy or HIV for example, and the person is potentially 'discreditable', they have to decide whether to be open about their condition or try to 'pass' as 'normal.' Thus the implications of stigma go well beyond public reaction. For example, Scambler and Hopkins (1986) found that very few of the epileptics they interviewed had actually experienced any stigmatising reactions from others (enacted stigma). However, the shame of being epileptic (felt stigma) led most of them to conceal their condition, even from those close to them. For example, two thirds of those experiencing epilepsy at the time of their marriage concealed it from their partners, while three-quarters had not disclosed their condition to their employers. The authors found that, paradoxically, this felt stigma was more disruptive to their lives than enacted stigma.

Managing stigma is therefore an important part of managing illness. However, being officially diagnosed and labelled is not necessarily stigmatising. Sometimes a diagnosis can have the opposite effect, For example, some conditions such as Parkinson's disease and multiple sclerosis can develop very slowly and there may be a long time between initial experiences of symptoms and medical diagnosis. In such circumstances diagnosis can be a relief as it both legitimises the patient's complaints and confirms the reality of their symptoms, while failure to obtain a diagnostic label can be stigmatising. In her study of encephalomyelitis (ME) Cooper (1997) found a great deal of conflict between patients who felt ill and their doctors who could find no evidence of disease. Consequently, many were not allowed access to the sick role and, as a result, 'their social position was to some extent eroded, their social identity devalued and stigmatised, and they found it difficult to obtain absence from work or disability benefit'.

Illness and identity

A great deal of the sociological research on experiences of illness comes from an interpretive approach in sociology called interactionism. A key area in interactionist sociology is the way in which people's self-concepts are developed over time through social relationships. People have the capacity to 'take the role of the other' and see themselves as they believe others see them. From this basis, interactionists are interested in the relationship between social reactions to illness and disability and individuals' self-concept and subsequent behaviour. Most of the earlier studies focused on the 'crisis' brought about by a person's comparatively sudden transition from 'health' to 'sickness' (Kelly & Field 1998). Some studies suggested that societal reaction creates a self-fulfilling prophecy where, though a process of socialisation, the person's identity comes to correspond to the meaning that others give to the condition.

Scott's (1969) classical study of the newly blind provides a good example of this approach. Scott argues that there is nothing inherent in the condition of blindness itself to produce the stereotyped view of the 'blind personality' as passive, docile and compliant. From his observations of interactions between experts and their blind clients, Scott argued that the 'blind personality' is a product of socialisation where experts emphasise to clients the importance of coming to terms with lost sight and accepting themselves as blind. This 'putative identity' is gradually internalised by clients as a basis for their own identity. Thus, according to Scott, blindness is a 'learned social role' because experts create for blind people the experience of being blind. Similarly, in his classic study of mental illness Scheff (1966) argued that mental hospitals socialise patients into playing a 'mentally ill role' (See Chapter 8).

More recent interactionist studies have tended to move from a 'crisis model' to a 'negotiation model', looking at illness more in terms of a series of gradual transformations of identity and experience. This change arose as a result of sociologists' increasing interest in chronic illnesses, such as arthritis, multiple sclerosis and Parkinson's disease, that develop slowly and inconsistently (Chapter 7). Chronic illness, for many people, is experienced as a series of status transitions. New ways of living and changes in self-concept have to be negotiated and re-negotiated as the disease progresses and sufferers have to readjust their patterns of work, leisure and personal relationships. Bury (1997) argues that in this 'negotiation model', illness is much more a *series* of adaptations to illness rather than the single adoption of an illness identity.

Adaptation to long-term illness involves managing both its physical and psychological aspects. The management of the physical aspects involves the development of new skills, such as operating machinery, administering medication and learning new daily routines. For example, sufferers from debilitating conditions, such as respiratory disorders, have to learn very quickly what they can do before chronic fatigue sets in and plan their day accordingly. The management of the physical aspects of illness is well described by Parsons' notion of the sick role, where people can be seen to be conforming to the 'obligations' involved in being ill. Psychological adaptation refers to the ways that people with chronic illness try to make sense of what Bury (1982) has called the 'biographical disruption' of their lives and identities. Part of this process involves people developing their own 'explanations' for the onset of the illness and its progression. Williams *et al.* (1996) showed how people with rheumatoid arthritis engage in a 'narrative reconstruction' in which their biography is reorganised in order to 'make sense' of the onset of illness. Narratives may also be used to explain sudden fluctuations in symptoms, such as having had a stressful experience, or 'overdoing things' the day before. While these 'lay theories' and 'narrative reconstructions' may have little or no clinical validity, they are often crucial in helping people restore a sense of order and meaning to their lives. As a result of this sociological work, health professionals have become much more interested in illness narratives, as they give insights into the patients' world and can lead to better professional–patient/client communication.

Nurse–patient relationships

So far, we have considered illness and illness management in general terms. However, nurse–patient relationships, like doctor–patient relationships, are influenced by a number of factors and can take different forms. Following Szasz and Hollander (1956), we can identify a continuum in the relative control exercised by nurses and patients over their interactions (Table 2.2). At one extreme, epitomised by intensive care settings, nurses are dominant and active while patients are passive and compliant. At the other extreme, found where nurses are employed to care for rich clients in their own home, the patient is dominant and the nurse responsive to their requirements. In between these extremes are situations where nurses guide alert and co-operative patients, for example in the treatment of infectious diseases

Table 2.2   Variations in nurse–patient relationships.

Nurse–patient	Nurse's role	Patient's role	Example
Active – Passive	Does something to the patient	Does what is told (may be hospital in-patient)	Coronary care nursing
Guidance – Co-operation	Tells patient what to do	Co-operates (obeys)	Acute infections
Mutual participation	Helps patients to help themselves	Negotiates treatment and other decisions with nurse	Most chronic illness, in the community
Co-operation – Guidance	Co-operates with patient in reaching the patient's goal(s)	Advises nurse what to do	Stable complex chronic disease managed at home
Passive – Active	Is told what to do by patient	Directs nurse	Rich patient receiving private nursing care

Source   Adapted from T.S. Szasz & M. Hollander (1956) A contribution to the philosophy of medicine, *AMA Archives of Internal Medicine*, xcvii, 585–92.

or accidental injuries, more equal relationships where nurse and patient help each other in the management of relatively stable long-term conditions, and even cases where knowledgeable patients guide nurses in the management of their condition. Primary nursing aims to move nurse–patient relationships to these more equal and co-operative patterns.

Disease conditions and places of care

The nature of the patient's disease condition has an important effect upon nurse–patient relationships. Where it develops slowly over a period of time, patients may have already made some adjustments to it, or mentally rehearsed possible outcomes of seeking professional help for it. With a sudden onset, particularly if it is as a result of an accident, there is no such preparation time, and the patient may be more dependent upon professional definitions. Where a condition is chronic but stable, the patient may become more expert in both its technical management and in recognising signs of deterioration or danger than the nurse, and hence take the lead role in its management.

The place where nurses and patients meet is another important factor influencing the relative power and control exercised by each party. Patients are likely to have the most control and influence in their own home (where the nurse is in some sense a guest) and least power and control as in-patients in an NHS hospital.

The nature of the condition and the places where nurses and patients meet seem the most powerful factors in producing the variations in 'activity' and 'passivity' suggested by Szasz and Hollander. Nurses (and other health professionals) are most powerful, active and controlling in hospital situations where the patient is critically ill and literally dependent upon their actions, whereas patients are most powerful, active and in control when the consultation is in their own homes and is about a long-standing, well-managed physical condition. However, nurse–patient relationships are also influenced by a number of other factors, such as the personal characteristics of the patient and the nurse, the relative knowledge each has about the condition and its treatment, and the social status and cultural background of patient and nurse.

'Good' and 'bad' patients

The ideas that nurses have about diseases and about patients influence their relationships with patients. Although the personal characteristics of patients and practitioners are not supposed to intrude into or influence treatment, the evidence is that they do have some effect upon relationships (for both doctors and nurses), and that they may influence patient care. It has been argued that 'good' patients, whose conditions challenge and expand nursing skills, tend to receive more care and attention than 'bad' patients, such as those with 'trivial' conditions or who are mutilated, incontinent or chronically or terminally ill. Patient behaviour is also influential, with co-operative, responsive patients who follow the rules being seen as 'good', while non-compliant, demanding, aggressive, complaining and manipulative patients are liable to be seen as 'bad'. However, Johnson and Webb (1995) suggest that while nurses do make social judgements about their patients it is difficult to make such broad generalisations. Nurses' evaluations may vary through time, they are usually aware of their labelling of patients, and to summarise their judgements in terms of 'good' and 'bad' patients oversimplifies complex behaviour.

Information and communication

What people know and understand about their condition is important, both for their well-being and for nurse–patient relationships. A recurrent finding in surveys of patient satisfaction with care is the dissatisfaction of patients with the information and communication they receive from health staff. To the extent that nurses and patients share the same views about the condition and its treatment, communication between them will be facilitated. However, where patients hold widely different views from nurses this may introduce conflict and tension into their relationship. It is in the latter situation that mis-communication and difficulties in assessing what information patients want are most likely to be found.

Nurses, like doctors, may try to maintain their control over patients by limiting or concealing information, especially in situations where there is 'bad news' for the patient. Research in the area of terminal care suggests that it is very difficult for nurses to conceal bad news from patients over any length of time, and that attempts to do so not only typically result in failure, but may also generate suspicion, mistrust, anger and hostility among patients. This has negative consequences for relationships between nurses and their patients (Chapter 9). With patient-centred nursing it is difficult to see how nurses' control of information in this manner can be justified. Where communication is free and open more trusting relationships are likely to be the norm and nurses are more likely to be able to respond to what patients want to know, to the benefit of all concerned.

Summary

The bio-medical model of health focuses on how the human body works and disease can be prevented, arrested or cured through treatment. Bio-medicine continues to dominate the organisation of health care in contemporary societies, but the capacity of a medically based health care system to influence overall patterns of health significantly is being increasingly questioned. A greater number of health professionals are now engaging in surveillance medicine, monitoring general populations with the idea of preventing disease and promoting better health. In the management of illness the bio-medical model is confined to the body and physical symptoms, but sociologists have shown that becoming ill also involves changes in social status and identity. Experiences of illness are shaped by the reactions of others and being ill involves processes of negotiation and narrative reconstruction. Nursing the sick involves the management of the social as well as the physical aspects of illness, although the scope and nature of nurse–patient relationships are influenced by a variety of factors and take different forms.

References

Anderson, D. (1991) The health activists: educators or propagandists? In: *Health, Lifestyle & Environment: countering the panic.* The Social Affairs Unit, Manhattan Institute.

Armstrong, D. (1995) The rise of surveillance medicine. *Sociology of Health and Illness,* **17**, 393–404.

Baggot, R. (1994) *Health and Health Care in Britain.* Palgrave, Basingstoke.

Berkman, L. & Syme, S. (1979) Social networks and host resistance and mortality: a nine year follow-up study of Almeda County residents. *American Journal of Epidemiology,* **109**, 186–204.

Bunker, J. (2001) Medicine matters after all. In: *Health and Disease: a reader,* 3rd edn. (eds B. Davey, A. Gray & C. Seale). Open University Press, Buckingham.

Bury, M. (1982) Chronic illness as biographical disruption. *Sociology of Health and Illness,* **4**, 167–82.

Bury, M. (1997) *Health and Illness in a Changing Society.* Routledge, London.

Cooper, L. (1997) Myalgic encephalomyelitis and the medical encounter. *Sociology of Health and Illness,* **19**, 186–207.

Durkheim, E. (1952) *Suicide.* Routledge, London.

Ell, K. (1996) Social networks, social support and coping with serious illness. *Social Science and Medicine,* **42**, 173–83.

Goffman, E. (1990) *Stigma: Notes on the Management of Spoiled Identity.* Penguin, London.

Graham, H. (1994) Gender and class as dimensions of smoking behaviour in Britain: insights from a survey of mothers. *Social Science and Medicine,* **38**, 691–8.

Graham, H. (ed.) (2000) *Understanding Health Inequalities.* Open University Press, Buckingham.

Hansell, P., Hughes, C., Caliandro, G., Russo, P., Budin, W., Hartman, B., Hernandez, O. (1998) The effect of a social support boosting intervention on stress, coping and social support in caregivers of children with HIV/AIDS. *Nursing Research,* **47**, 79–86.

Illich, I. (1990) *Limits to Medicine: Medical Nemesis: The Expropriation of Health.* Penguin, London.

Jeffrey, R. (2001) Normal rubbish: deviant patients in casualty departments. In: *Health and Disease: a reader*, 3rd edn. (eds B. Davey, A. Gray & C. Seale). Open University Press, Buckingham.

Johnson, M. & Webb, C. (1995) Rediscovering the unpopular patient: the concept of social judgement. *Journal of Advanced Nursing*, **21**, 466–75.

Kelly, M. (1996) *A Code of Ethics for Health Promotion*. Social Affairs Unit, London.

Kelly, M. & Field, D. (1998) Conceptualising Chronic Illness. In: *Sociological Perspectives on Health, Illness and Health Care* (eds D. Field & S. Taylor). Blackwell, Oxford.

Le Fanu, J. (1999) *The Rise and Fall of Modern Medicine*. Little, Brown & Co., London.

Macleod Clark, J. (1993) From sick nursing to health nursing: evolution or revolution? In: *Research in Health Promotion and Nursing* (eds J. Wilson-Barnet & J. Macleod Clark). Palgrave, Basingstoke.

McKeown, T. (1979) *The Role of Medicine*. Blackwell, Oxford.

McKinlay, J. & McKinlay, S. (1977) The questionable contribution of medical measures to the decline of mortality in the United States in the twentieth century. *Milbank Memorial Fund Quarterly*, **55**, 405–28.

Medical Services Study Group of the Royal College of Physicians of London (1978) Deaths under 50. *British Medical Journal*, **2**, 1061–2.

Nyamathi, A., Leake, B., Keenan, C., Gelberg, L. (2000) Type of social support among homeless women: its impact on psychosocial resources, health and health behaviours and use of services. *Nursing Research*, **49**, 318–26.

Oliver, M. (1996) *Understanding Disability: From Theory to Practice*. Palgrave, Basingstoke.

Parsons, T. (1951) *The Social System*. Free Press, New York.

Reinharz, S. (2001) Enough already! The pervasiveness of warnings in everyday life. In: *Health and Disease: a reader*, 3rd edn. (eds B. Davey, A. Gray & Seale). Open University Press, Buckingham.

Scambler, G. & Hopkins, A. (1986) Being epileptic: coming to terms with illness. *Sociology of Health and Illness*, **8**, 26–43.

Scheff, T. (1966) *Being Mentally Ill: a Sociological Theory*. Aldine, Chicago.

Scott, R. (1969) *The Making of Blind Men*. Russell Sage, Hartford. Conn.

Seale, C., Pattison, S. & Davey, B. (eds) (2001) *Medical Knowledge: Doubt and Certainty*. Open University Press, Buckingham.

Secretary of State for Health and Social Services (1992) *The Health of the Nation*. HMSO, London.

Szasz, T. & Hollander, M. (1956) A contribution to the philosophy of medicine. *AMA Archives of Internal Medicine*, **xcvii**, 585–92.

Szreter, S. (1988) The importance of social intervention in Britain's mortality decline. *Social History of Medicine*, **1**, 1–38.

Taylor, S. & Tilley, N. (1989) Health visitors and child protection: conflict, contradictions and ethical dilemmas. *Health Visitor*, **62**, 273–5.

Turner, B. (1995) *Medical Power and Social Knowledge*. Sage, London.

Wadsworth, M., Butterfield, W. & Blaney, R. (1971) *Health and Sickness: The Choice of Treatment*, Tavistock, London.

Williams, G., Fitzpatrick, R., MacGregor, A. & Rigby, A. (1996) Rheumatoid arthritis. In: *Experiencing and Explaining Disease* (eds B. Davey & C. Seale). Open University Press, Buckingham.

Williams, S. & Calnan, M. (1996) The 'limits' of demedicalisation: modern medicine and the lay populace in 'late' modernity. *Social Science and Medicine*, **42**, 609–20.

Further reading

Davey, B., Gray, A. & Seale, C. (eds) (2001) *Health and Disease: a reader*, 3rd edn. Open University Press, Buckingham.

Seale, C., Pattison, S. & Davey, B. (eds) (2001) *Medical Knowledge: Doubt and Certainty*. Open University Press, Buckingham.

Part II
Social Patterns in Health and Disease

Chapter 3
Socio-economic Inequalities in Health

Inequalities in health between social groups are an extremely resilient feature of British society and continue to be part of the social and political landscape of the early twenty-first century. Although the associations between poverty and health have been recognised for over 150 years, until quite recently research was severely hampered by the twin problems of political indifference to health inequalities and the absence of complete and reliable data. Fortunately today, health professionals are able to draw upon a wealth of research to explore the complex relationship between people's health and their socio-economic circumstances. This chapter will provide an overview of the evidence about socio-economic inequalities in health and the explanations of these. It will:

- Discuss the measurement of socio-economic status and health
- Review the historical background of contemporary health inequalities
- Discuss the widening gap in socio-economic health inequalities
- Examine explanations of socio-economic health inequalities
- Consider what might be done to reduce socio-economic health inequalities

Measuring inequality and health

Before we look at the evidence we will briefly consider how researchers have measured socio-economic status and health.

Socio-economic status

This measure is associated with the sociological conceptualisation of social class, first proposed by Marx. The concept of social class is most frequently measured by the indicator of occupational ranking (Chapter 1). Socio-economic status is a wider concept than social class, referring to an array of factors such as income level, education, housing, power, and social status. A number of these are often combined to produce a composite measure.

Occupation is the foundation of the widely used British Registrar General's measure of social class, which has been in use since 1921. Until recently the schema was based on five groups defined by occupational skill (depicted in Table 3.1 and Table 3.3). It has recently been revised in a new version to take account of labour market changes such as the increase in information technology, service sector work, and remote service work (e.g. homeworking and Call Centre employment). This new version is called the National Statistics Socio-economic Classification (or NS-SEC) and came into use with the 2001 Census. While the previous classification suffered from the inability to account for those not in employment – such as people who have never worked, are retired, and welfare recipients – the current classification covers all the adult population. Since this classification is very new at the time of writing, it is not possible to include research evidence based on its use here. However, it will be in use, especially when data from the 2001 Census is available and it is likely to be at the heart of British research for the foreseeable future.

Some researchers are unhappy with the use of occupation as the measure of socio-economic status. It has been argued that we now live in a society defined as much by consumption and status as by work and production. For this reason, measures such as home ownership, car ownership, income and deprivation are sometimes preferred. Importantly, these measures also allow us to examine differences *within* occupationally defined groups, and provide a more detailed analysis of health and mortality. For example, people's lives are significantly shaped by the places in which they live and indeed the characteristics of their area of residence may have a greater effect on their health than personal characteristics such as occupation. For this reason deprivation indices, based on small area statistics from the Census have been used for many years. Indeed, much recent research on inequality in health has been geographically based using such measures. For example, in 1999 Shaw *et al.* produced a geographical analysis of parliamentary constituencies throughout Britain.

Health

Although it may seem rather strange to use death as a measure of health, mortality statistics are the most reliable way of measuring health inequalities. Most importantly, since they have been available for many years, we can reliably track changes over time. However, age at death and the causes of death tell us relatively little about the experience of health and illness during life. Capturing the experience of health and illness, and relating it to inequality is difficult because the way that people define their health is subjective and can itself be influenced by their socio-economic status (Blane 1998). Researchers use a large number of different indicators to try to measure morbidity or illness and consistent socio-economic differences in health have been found by most of these measures of morbidity. Researchers have found that the simple overall self-assessment of health as 'good' or 'bad' is usually the single best predictor of health status. At the present time, the most frequently used measures in official surveys such as the decennial Census and the annual General Household Survey (GHS) are self-reported prevalence of long-standing illness, and global self-assessments of overall health.

Historical background

Despite massive social change and improvement in the overall health of the nation, little has been achieved in reducing the health gap between rich and poor since the

1800s. Not only do the patterns of inequality seem familiar, but also current explanations for them strongly echo more than century-old debates. For example, recent emphasis on individual responsibility for ill-health parallels debate in the 1800s about whether poverty and related ill-health arose from 'the failings of individuals or from the failings of society' (Davey Smith *et al.* 2001). Questions of whether poverty causes ill-health or ill-health causes poverty also stem back to this time. Arguments for the foundation of the NHS (established in 1948) gave considerable emphasis to poverty and lack of access to health care. We can also see continuity between the eugenics movement of the early twentieth century, which stressed that heredity had a greater influence upon health than social environment, and present day socio-biological and genetic accounts for differences in health (Davey Smith *et al.* 2001)

Influential research from the middle of the twentieth century added new insights showing that, despite increasing affluence, social equality had grown considerably and suggesting that although a society as a whole could get both richer and healthier, health inequalities between people could actually increase in the process. By the 1970s the accumulated research was sufficient to suggest that many Britons were experiencing an undue burden of ill-health and that persisting health inequalities might be contributing to this. The Black Report, published in 1980 (Townsend *et al.* 1988) reviewed this evidence and concluded that 'the predominant or governing explanation for inequalities in health [lies] in material deprivation' and proposed a comprehensive anti-poverty strategy to address this. However, this did not match up with the thinking of the incoming Conservative government of 1979 which placed less emphasis on societal factors and more on personal responsibility for health, wealth and opportunity. This view prevailed for two decades.

During its period in opposition, the Labour Party criticised the Conservative government's failure to implement the recommendations of the Black Report and when it came into power in 1997 it set up a new inquiry into health inequality. This endorsed the Black Report's conclusion that the origins of health inequalities lie in the social environment and concluded that, even though the previous twenty years had brought a marked increase in prosperity to the country as a whole, the gap between the top and bottom social strata had widened at all stages of the lifecourse, reflected in growing inequalities in health (Acheson Report 1998).

The widening gap in socio-economic health inequalities

Research subsequent to the publication of the Black Report has confirmed a consistent relationship between socio-economic inequalities and ill-health. The authors of the Black Report were forced to rely on mortality figures in their analysis of health inequalities because there were very little population-level data available that tracked patterns of health – as opposed to death – over time. In the intervening period there has been a massive expansion of research on ill-health and inequality but, since most data on health status cannot be reliably collected retrospectively, our access to data which looks at changes in health over long time-periods is still rather limited.

Mortality

Figure 3.1 displays the widening mortality gap over time between people at the 'top' and the 'bottom' of the social hierarchy in simple diagrammatic terms. It shows that the gap is widening because even though mortality rates are improving across the board, the rate of improvement has been faster among those at the 'top', than among those at the 'bottom'.

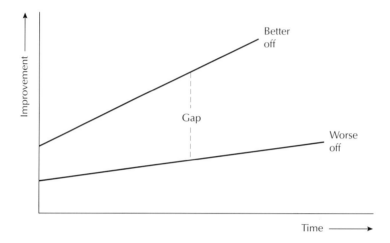

Fig. 3.1　The widening mortality gap.

The figures in Table 3.1 highlight this change. They show that mortality rates have clearly declined – that is, improved – for both men and women between the two periods, but the gap between those in 'professional/managerial' and those in 'partly skilled and unskilled' occupations, has grown. The ratio of 'top' to 'bottom', displayed at the foot of the table, shows that in the late 1970s, death rates were 53% higher among men at the 'bottom' than among men at the 'top'. By the late 1980s this difference had increased to 68%. There are similar differences among women,

Table 3.1　Age-standardised[1] mortality rates per 100 000 people, selected years, women and men aged 35–64, England and Wales. Crown copyright.

	1976–81		1986–92	
	Women	Men	Women	Men
I/II Professional/managerial	338	621	270	455
IIIN Skilled (non-manual)	371	860	305	484
IIIM Skilled (manual)	467	802	356	624
IV/V Partly skilled/unskilled	508	951	418	764
Ratio of I/II:IV/V	*1.50*	*1.53*	*1.55*	*1.68*

[1] Age-standardisation adjusts for the effects of any differences in the age distribution of different occupational class groups.
Source　Adapted from *The Acheson Report* (1998) Table 3. (Stationery Office)

although they are much less marked. Death rates among women at the 'bottom' were 50% higher than those at the 'top' in the late 1970s, and 55% higher in the late 1980s. Gender differences in health are discussed in Chapter 5 of this book.

Another useful indicator of health inequality is potential life lost, i.e. the number of years earlier than the average life expectancy that people die. There were just over twice as many years of potential life lost among men aged between 20 and 64 in 'unskilled', compared to 'professional' occupations in the early 1970s. This had risen to over three times as many years lost by the early 1990s (Blane & Drever 1998).

Morbidity

Although the population of Britain are living longer, these years are not necessarily spent in good health. For example, the numbers of people reporting either long-standing or short-term illnesses in the GHS have shown no overall improvement since the 1970s. It seems that worsening health among those in poorer socio-economic circumstances may be contributing to this, leading Davey Smith (1996) to suggest that 'inequality may make people miserable long before it kills them'.

Table 3.2 presents data on levels of permanent sickness by the areas in which people live (here defined by parliamentary constituencies) from the 1981 and 1991 Censuses of the population. Permanent sickness, as defined in the Census, refers to being 'unable to work because of long-term sickness or disability'. These data show that the percentage increases in permanent sickness between 1981 and 1991 were much larger in the 'least healthy' than in the 'most healthy areas'. Importantly, the 'worst health' areas also tend to be areas of higher socio-economic deprivation, as measured by a range of factors. For example, the 'worst health' areas have a higher percentage of people living in poverty, higher unemployment levels, and lower average incomes than the 'best health' areas (Shaw *et al.* 1999). In his Annual Report for 2001 the Chief Medical Officer for Health highlighted that as recently as the late 1990s some of the 'worst off' communities in England – such as central Manchester,

Table 3.2 People with permanent sickness and unable to work, over age 15 in Britain (1981 and 1991).

Area	Number in 1991	% in 1981	% in 1991	Increase
'Worst health areas'				
Glasgow Shettleston	5663	4	12	3370
Liverpool Riverside	6576	4	11	3332
Salford	5153	4	8	2399
Manchester Blackley	5440	3	8	2888
'Best health areas'				
South Norfolk	1743	2	2	647
Northavon	1598	2	2	482
Buckingham	1094	2	2	236

Source M. Shaw *et al.* (1999) *The Widening Gap. Health Inequalities and Policy in Britain*. Selected data from Table 4.9.

and Manvers in Nottingham – had death rates equivalent to the national average back in 1950. This reflects the intense concentration of poverty in inner city areas.

Trends for a different measure of health – self-reported long-standing illness – show that its prevalence (measured by occupation, as shown in Table 3.1) has been consistently worse for those in manual, compared to those in non-manual groups. Over the period 1979 to 1994, the ratio of long-standing illness between 'top' and 'bottom' was consistently about 1.5:1 for men, and nearly 2:1 for women. This suggests that, in contrast to permanent sickness (which is a narrower way of measuring illness) the socio-economic health gap in long-standing illness is unchanged. There is even some evidence that the gap may be gradually declining among women (Bunting 1997).

Given their impact upon health, it is also important to consider the distribution of 'health behaviours' such as diet, exercise and cigarette smoking within the population. Because there is reliable data available over time, cigarette smoking can be used as an example. Although overall smoking rates have declined over time, the differential between the highest and lowest occupational groups widened considerably between 1974 and 1994. There was some fluctuation for men, but in 1974 those in the unskilled manual group were just over twice as likely to smoke as those in the professional group. By 1994, this had increased to a two and a half-fold differential. The widening gap is even more marked for women. In 1974 the unskilled manual group were nearly twice as likely to smoke as women in the professional group, by 1994 the difference had increased to nearly three times (Bunting 1997).

Since health and illness can be measured in a number of ways it is not surprising to find that by some measures we see an increasing socio-economic gap, while for others we see stability. The most important point is the consistent finding that at *any one point in time*, those at the top of the social hierarchy are in much better health than those at the bottom. We can see this in a range of current data. For a final example, Table 3.3 depicts significant differences in self-assessed general health by socio-economic status. The gradients are remarkably clear: as we go down the socio-economic hierarchy (here measured by the social class of the 'head of household'), both men's and women's assessments of their own health consistently worsen.

Table 3.3 Adults' self-assessed general health (%) (age-standardised). Adults age 19 and over, 1996. Crown copyright.

	Good/very good		Fair		Bad/very bad	
	Men	Women	Men	Women	Men	Women
I Professional	87	87	11	11	2	3
II Employers/managers	85	80	12	16	3	4
IIIN Skilled (non-manual)	81	78	13	16	5	5
IIIM Skilled (manual)	74	72	19	22	7	6
IV Partly skilled/personal service	72	69	19	23	9	7
V Unskilled manual	67	65	25	29	9	5

Source *Health Survey for England 1996*, Vol 1 (DoH 1998). Adaptation of Table 5.14.

Explanations for socio-economic health inequalities

Access to health care

One explanation that has prevailed for a long time is that socio-economic differences in health reflect differences in access to health care. Indeed, back in the 1940s it was assumed that removing financial barriers to access to the NHS would promote more equitable care and thus improve the health of the worse-off in society. However, the picture is quite complicated. This is reflected in patterns of use by socio-economic status. Recent GHS (ONS 2001) data shows that people in lower socio-economic groups are more likely to have consulted a GP in the 14 days before the interview. However for the large majority of age groups, the difference is not statistically significant. General practice is important since it is typically the 'gatekeeper' to other more specialist services, but it is only the tip of the iceberg of the wider range of services (e.g. primary care, hospital care, preventative and screening services, maternity care, diagnostic services and so on) for a variety of health problems. Examination of the evidence about access to this wider range of health services does not reveal a consistent picture of worse access for lower socio-economic groups (Goddard & Smith 2001).

We also need to bear in mind that even if use *were* equal, this would not necessarily mean that health care needs were being equally met. As we have seen, people in worse-off socio-economic circumstances tend to have worse health which means that their *need* is typically greater. In discussions of health service use this is often called the *demand side* of the equation and research often points to a reservoir of *unmet need*. There is also the *supply side* of service use. This refers to the kind of services that are delivered. Back in 1971 Tudor Hart outlined the 'inverse care law' which describes a situation in which people in deprived areas tend to have greater health care needs, but that services are much less likely to be available (and may be of a poorer quality) (Arblaster & Hastings 2000). This persists today and has been the subject of longstanding policy initiatives such as the provision of deprivation payments to general practice/Primary Care Teams in deprived areas and, since the late 1990s, the classification of deprived areas as Health Action Zones.

Overall, factors on both the demand and supply side suggest that there may be socio-economic inequalities in access to health care. However it is important to remember that increases in life expectancy between the mid-eighteenth and midtwentieth century were more to do with improvements in the social and economic environment than developments in medicine, suggesting that health care has a limited role in explaining the health of the population in general (Chapter 2). For these reasons, while health care may play a role, it is unlikely to be the major explanation for inequalities in health. Social scientists have therefore turned their attention to the wider socio-economic environments in which people live.

Explanations in the Black Report

The authors of the Black Report of 1980 (Townsend *et al.* 1988) reviewed the three main explanations of socio-economic inequalities in health that were current at the time. The first explanation, which they favoured, was that differences in health are socially caused by differences in *material (economic) circumstances* such as income, housing, and working environment; those in worse material conditions have worse health as a result. An opposite argument is called *social (or health) selection*. Here the direction of causation is reversed: it is not material circumstances that influence levels of health and illness, but, rather, levels of health and illness that influence material circumstances. People are *selected* into social positions on the basis of their health; for example, those in poor health are unlikely to hold on to well-paid jobs and are liable to move down the occupational ladder, while those with good health are more likely to be upwardly mobile. Higher social classes tend to recruit the healthiest individuals, while the least healthy 'fall' into the lower classes. The third explanation the Black Report focused on was differences in *cultures and behaviours* between social classes. People in the lower social classes are more likely to define health as the absence of symptoms and to have low expectations of health, seeing illness as a matter of luck or fate. People from professional and managerial backgrounds have higher expectations about health, believing that their own behaviour can improve it, share medical definitions of health and illness, and are more likely to seek expert help at an early stage in their illness. These different health beliefs are related to differences in health behaviour – such as smoking, exercise, diet – between higher (better informed, with healthier behaviour) and lower (ill-informed, with unhealthy behaviour) social classes.

Layers of influence

Following the Black Report, explanations of health inequality in the 1980s tended to pit structural factors that affect health which are largely outside the individual's control, such as pollution, levels of unemployment, and access to health care, against factors over which they have somewhat more control, such as diet and exercise. Government health policy of the time emphasised that 'unhealthy behaviours' which contribute to ill-health, such as smoking and eating foods high in sugar and fat, predominated in working class households. Following on from this, Government health improvement policies predominantly focused on changing individual behaviour, rather than the wider social environment. However, academic debate was increasingly stressing the *interaction* of structural factors and individual behaviours, for example that living in an area of high unemployment and being unable to find work causes stress which in turn provokes unhealthy behaviours like cigarette smoking. This kind of approach is endorsed in the Acheson Report (1998) which depicts the main determinants of health as layers of influence, one over another (Fig. 3.2).

  At the centre of the model are individuals who 'are endowed with age, sex, and constitutional factors which undoubtedly influence health potential, but are relatively fixed' (Acheson Report 1998). The innermost layer represents individual lifestyle factors such as diet and exercise. The next layer recognises that 'individuals do not exist in a vacuum: they interact with friends, relatives and their immediate community' and this influences their health in both positive and negative ways. The third, outer layer, depicts the wider socio-economic, cultural and

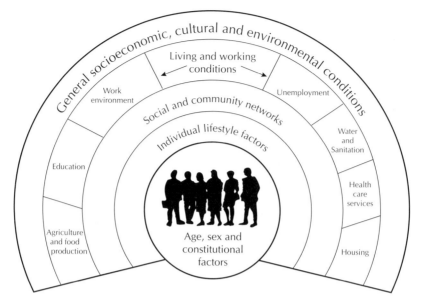

Fig. 3.2 Social determinants of health.
Source The Acheson Report, 1998, crown copyright.

environmental conditions which influence a person's ability to maintain their health such as their work environment, housing and the availability of health care.

Understanding health inequalities involves tracing the paths between layers, from outside inwards and inside outwards. Or, to put it another way, exploring how the socio-economic structure of society influences individuals and how individuals influence the socio-economic structure. The remainder of this section will use this model to discuss the influence of general socio-economic factors: the role of social and community networks, individual lifestyle and the lifecourse, and the 'psychosocial pathways' between socio-economic status and health.

General socio-economic factors

Large-scale quantitative research has been most successful in tracing the paths that run from social structure to the individual, that is, from 'outside-in'. In particular, it has demonstrated the strong association between changes in health and the dynamics of socio-economic circumstances (the outer layer in Fig. 3.2) over time. It is therefore important to review the kinds of changes that have been occurring.

Graham (2000) neatly sums up recent socio-economic change as follows, 'during the 1980s and 1990s greater prosperity for the majority has been at the cost of poverty for an increasing minority'. Figure 3.3 shows changes in household incomes in the United Kingdom (adjusted to April 1999 prices) since the early 1970s. During the 1970s, household income at the top, middle and bottom of the income scale rose at more or less the same pace. Significant changes began in the 1980s. While

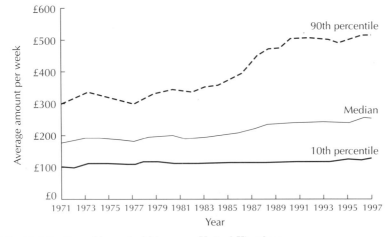

Fig. 3.3 Distribution of household income, United Kingdom.
Source F. Prever *et al.* (2000) *Social Inequalities* 2000 edition. The Stationery Office, London.

incomes rose on average for everyone, the gap between top and bottom began to increase: as the income for the top 10% of households rose by 38%; the income for those in the middle (the median) rose by about 25%; and the income of the bottom 10% rose by only 5%. Although there was greater stability during the 1990s, it is notable that even during this period the household income of the top tenth was about four times higher than the bottom tenth. This is a much larger difference than the start of the 1970s, when the equivalent difference was just over threefold (Drever *et al.* 2000).

The official definition of relative poverty is an income below 60% of the population median (i.e. the mid point). At the start of the 1980s, this accounted for less than 15% of the population, but this rose steadily throughout the 1980s to stabilise during the 1990s at around 24% (Drever *et al.* 2000). Many researchers have pointed out that these inequalities are driven by significant changes in patterns of employment in contemporary Britain with more part-time, temporary and flexible work, more self-employment and more long-term chronic unemployment. To return to the terminology used above, this suggests that the pathways 'outside in' are built upon a foundation of growing income inequality based on the changing economic structure of modern Britain.

These kinds of change in socio-economic conditions have been strongly associated with the widening gap in health inequalities documented earlier in the chapter. Indeed, for some researchers they provide *the* most compelling explanation for them (e.g. Shaw *et al.* 1999). However, others have pointed out that this may be an overly deterministic view that 'all too readily creates a picture of "the poor", "the working class" ... as victims of circumstance' (Bury 1997). In terms of the 'layers of influence model' (Fig. 3.2), explanations which propose socio-economic change as the sole, or even major, explanatory factor, only take us so far since they cannot easily explain the pathways 'inside out', i.e. that people do not only follow paths dictated to them by wider socio-economic circumstances, they modify them, and even create their own.

Social and community networks, living and working conditions

Social and community networks are the meeting point between the socio-economic determinants of health (the employment opportunities, levels of deprivation and so on described above) and individual behaviours or 'lifestyle factors' that influence health. The question of which is more important, social environment or individual behaviour in determining health is probably impossible to answer (Blaxter 1990). This is because they are so closely bound together: individual lifestyles are likely to be rooted in and grow out of particular social contexts. Although there is substantial evidence that the way that people view their health, the decisions that they make about their health (such as whether to consult a doctor or not), and the health-promoting or health-damaging behaviours that they engage in are strongly associated with their socio-economic position, the fit is far from complete. After all, not all middle-class people are healthy and not all working-class people are unhealthy. Moreover, even if we find a strong *statistical association* between, say, being middle class and in good health, this tells us nothing about the complex social mechanisms – such as how people interpret and act on their circumstances – which actually link the two. It is in recognition of these points that social scientists now suggest that we should ground our analysis of health inequalities much more firmly in the social and community networks within which people live out their lives.

Important new and relatively unexplored research questions arise from this perspective such as, what are the health consequences of being an individual living in poor socio-economic circumstances in a relatively prosperous place? How do individuals who live in the most materially disadvantaged areas make sense of and act upon their environments, and with what consequences for health? (Blaxter 1990). It is still very early days in terms of turning these theoretical questions into empirical research that explores exactly how people and place interact. In this respect it is far more likely that answers will be found from in-depth qualitative research of individuals and their communities than large-scale statistical surveys.

Individual lifestyle and the life course

One way that researchers are exploring the link between health-related behaviours and social structures is through biographical research on the lifecourse. This not only illuminates the 'multiple and fluid social locations' that people occupy, but also how and why these change across time and place and their relevance for the lived experience of health (Popay & Groves 2000). Health status is a product of cumulative experiences built up over a lifetime. However, it is very difficult to know exactly how this occurs since much of the data on inequalities in health are snapshots in time. Even data which looks at trends over time is often not truly longitudinal as far as the individual is concerned. For example, the data in Table 3.1 and Table 3.2 do not follow-up the *same individuals* over time, but rather track changes in occupational social classes and in geographical areas at the aggregate level. Yet individuals have different experiences of health and their shared socio-economic environment, and these change over the lifecourse. Personal experiences are not static – although it may seem this way when they are conceptualised only in terms of broad socio-economic categories. For example changing a job (even within the same social class category), or moving to a new home (although in the same census area), may have significant impacts on health, as has been shown in research on the relationship between 'life events' and health (Chapter 2).

Individual biographies

The changes in individual lives over time can tell us a lot about how life experience impacts on health. As their lives unfold people develop certain understandings and expectations about their lives, often linked to their socio-economic circumstances, which relate to their health (Blaxter 2000). For example, different socio-economic groups may have different expectations of what counts as health and a healthy life (Blaxter 1990). These expectations may also affect how they interpret symptoms of disease and whether they seek help. There are expectations about how individual lives should proceed through *calendar time*. For example, in contemporary Britain children are not expected to die before their parents, and those who do are thought to have died 'before their time'. As Blaxter (2000) puts it, generally 'years go by at a regular pace in the lives of individuals, child following parent and adulthood following childhood'. Personal biographies are also embedded within what Blaxter calls *socio-historical time*. This refers to the experiences of people born into particular generations (age cohorts), each with their own unique social history. Different age-cohorts experience quite particular socio-economic vulnerabilities, such as those associated with employment conditions (e.g. the use of asbestos, leading to abestosis, which peaked in the 1970s) or medical knowledge (e.g. cigarette smoking was not widely known to be dangerous to health until the 1960s).

Research into the relationships between socio-economic status, individual life courses and health is a relatively new but increasingly important area of activity. Research on age-cohorts and generations and on the individual lifecourse is important in two ways. First, it helps us to understand how individual biographies are played out within their wider social context and the implications of this for health. Second, it provides insight into how the health of one generation builds on the health of the generation before it. This takes us to the role of biology in health inequalities.

The influence of biology

From a lifecourse perspective on health inequalities, a person's biological status is a marker of their past social position, recording a lifetime of accumulated advantage and disadvantage. Figure 3.4 summarises two main explanations of this socio-biological link between early life and adult disease.

The first explanation gives primacy to events *in utero* or in infancy that 'programme' the individual's ability to respond to risks to health that are encountered later in life. Although later life influences play a role, this is 'only within the constraints imposed by early development' (Power *et al* 1996). The second explanation highlights continuities in lifetime circumstances. Here 'biological' factors such as birth weight are to a degree caused by prior social factors such as parental social circumstances; low birth weight (LBW) then becomes a marker for later social

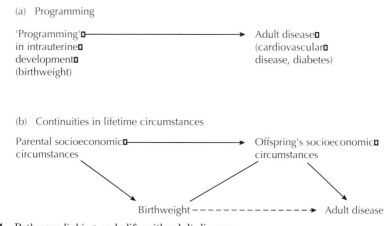

Fig. 3.4 Pathways linking early life with adult disease.
Source Power, C., Bartley, M., Davey Smith, G., & Blane, D. (1996) Transmission of Social and Biological Risk Across the lifecourse. *Health and Social Organisation* (eds D. Blane, R. Brunner & R. Wilkinson). Routledge, London. Reproduced with permission of Thompson Publishing, London.

disadvantage (such as poor educational attainment) and, consequently, poor health. As Wadsworth (1999) aptly puts it 'childhood has a long reach'.

Events begin *in utero*. Groundbreaking research by Barker and his colleagues highlighted the crucial impact of under-nutrition in middle to late gestation on health in later life. Direct associations have been made between LBW and increased rates of coronary heart disease (CHD) (Barker 1995). Physiologically it would seem that if the fetus experiences under-nutrition in late gestation, oxygenated blood is diverted from the trunk to sustain the brain. This affects the growth of the liver, in the process disturbing its regulation of cholesterol and blood clotting, both risk factors for CHD (Wadsworth 1999). All of this takes place in a social context, and age-cohort studies – such as the 1958 British birth cohort study – highlight that longer-term health is influenced by 'parental disadvantage and low birth weight; some or all of, financial hardship and poor nutrition, crowded residential accommodation and disrupted sleep patterns, and delayed growth during childhood; and the social circumstances which delay childhood growth predispose to labour market disadvantage, as indexed by prolonged or frequent spells in unemployment' (Blane 1999).

Thus, referring back to Fig. 3.4, it is not simply a matter of our future health being 'programmed' from birth, but rather of biology interacting with the social environment in which we live. As Wadsworth (1999) puts it, 'biological programming processes require a later-life additional risk to push individuals beyond their biologically programmed safe working envelope'. These additional risks – such as cigarette smoking and obesity – are themselves socially determined.

In this section we have explored the main determinants of health inequalities in terms of layers of influence one over another. It has been stressed that far from being competing explanations, structural or material factors, individual behaviours and biology interact to produce inequalities in health. The main question currently exercising researchers is exactly *how* this takes place. One of the most influential and much debated explanations is Richard Wilkinson's (1996) theory of the 'psychosocial pathways' between socio-economic status and health.

Relative deprivation and psychosocial stress

Wilkinson's (1996) thesis is that in contemporary societies such as Britain the psychosocial effects of living in conditions of *relative deprivation* are a more important influence upon people's health than *absolute material deprivation*. He argues that those who are in positions of relative deprivation have less autonomy and control over their lives, have weak social affiliations and experience more stress in their early life.

There are three key stages to his argument. First, he shows that for wealthy developed countries there is a threshold beyond which the absolute standard of living of the population is no longer associated with improvements in health, measured by life expectancy. He argues that once a country has passed through the epidemiological transition (i.e. the shift away from infectious to degenerative diseases as the major cause of death) 'its whole population can be more than twice as rich as any other country without being any healthier'. This suggests that there are clear limits on the health returns of a country getting more and more wealthy. Second, he argues that although the absolute standard of living is not important for wealthy societies like Britain, differences *within* society, such as differences in income, are crucial to health inequalities. That is, it is where individuals stand *in relation to others* (i.e. relative deprivation) that matters most. Third, he argues that the key mechanism linking relative deprivation to health is psychosocial. Simply put, as income differences widened in Britain during the 1980s (in the manner described earlier in the chapter), psychosocial stress increased and we saw a slow-down in the improvement in overall mortality rates.

This takes us back to the association between biology and health, and the changing socio-economic structure of societies such as Britain. Wilkinson argues that 'many of the biological processes that lead to ill-health are triggered by *what we think and feel* about our material and social circumstances' (Wilkinson 2000, my emphasis). It is therefore our subjective experience of life that is important. He argues that as individualism and the ethos of the market hold sway and civic morality declines, our health is compromised. Feelings of hopelessness, anxiety, insecurity and anger amongst those living in relative deprivation leave their mark upon health, directly through weakened immunity and indirectly through negative health-related behaviours such as smoking, and the consumption of alcohol and high-fat and high-sugar 'comfort foods'.

Wilkinson puts forward two kinds of evidence to demonstrate the importance of psychosocial pathways for health. The first concerns the relationship between income and health. Among developed countries, it is the most egalitarian that have the highest life expectancy, not the richest. This is because more egalitarian societies are more cohesive as seen, for example, in higher levels of trust between people. During World War II, Britain saw a rise in life expectancy among civilians alongside a narrowing of income differences and an increase in social cohesion, despite the fact that *absolute* economic circumstances declined for many people. A second example compares Britain and Japan. In 1970 the two countries were quite similar in terms of life expectancy and income distribution. Subsequently, the income distribution for Japan has narrowed considerably while life expectancy has increased quite dramatically to reach the highest recorded for any country reporting to the World Bank. By comparison, as we have seen, in Britain income differentials widened substantially over the 1980s and its ranking in the life expectancy league table fell.

The second kind of evidence comes from research into the physiological effects of social status among animals. In studies of macaque monkeys, it is possible to hold factors such as diet and environment (e.g. access to water, food and space), constant while manipulating social status. The research showed that animals in low-status groups developed very significant risks to health such as increased atherosclerosis (hardening of the arteries), unfavourable ratios of high-density lipoprotein cholesterol and low-density lipoprotein cholesterol, insulin resistance, and a tendency to central obesity.

The policy implication of Wilkinson's thesis is clear: a redistribution of wealth to create a more egalitarian and cohesive society will reduce health inequalities, by improving the health of the worse-off. He argues that 'every £1000 redistributed from rich to poor tends to improve the health of the poor more than its loss harms the health of the rich' (2000). This is not simply because average standards of health rise, but also because everyone tends to be healthier – whatever their income – in a more egalitarian society.

The main criticism of Wilkinson's thesis is that in attending to the 'psychosocial pathways' which link socio-economic status to health he fails to identify the *root cause* of health inequalities: absolute material deprivation *is* more important than relative psychosocial deprivation, and leads to the latter. In Coburn's view, it is not so much that income inequality produces lower cohesion and trust, leading to poor health, but that 'neo-liberalism (market dominance) produces both higher income inequality and lower social cohesion' (Coburn 2000). He continues that, in a neo-liberal market economy, where competition and individualism are valued above all, it is not surprising that we have seen a decline in community and trust between people. Lynch *et al.* (2000) broadly concur with this view, stressing that 'the structural, political-economic processes that generate inequality exist before their effects are experienced at the individual level'.

Addressing socio-economic health inequalities

The Acheson Report (1998) highlighted two general points: first, the origins of health inequality lie in the social environment; second, health inequalities are increasing. The new Labour Government endorsed these conclusions, named health inequalities as one of its top priorities and published a set of targets to tackle them (DoH 2001):

- To reduce by at least 10% the gap between the fifth of health authority areas with the lowest life expectancy at birth and the population as a whole by 2010
- To reduce by at least 10% the gap in infant mortality between manual groups and the population as a whole by 2010
- To reduce the number of children living in poverty by a quarter by 2004

- To reduce smoking rates among manual groups from 32% in 1998 to 26% by 2010
- To reduce teenage pregnancy (e.g. reducing the under-18 conception rate) by 15% by 2004 and 50% by 2010

It recognised that tackling health inequalities involves not only identifying targets, but also developing a strategy to deal with them.

There are no simple solutions to reducing socio-economic health inequalities because these are caused by a number of factors operating at different levels. Individual health behaviours have been a longstanding focus of government intervention, and an important part of nursing work, especially in the community, is focused on these. However, as we have seen in this chapter, people's health behaviours cannot be divorced from the effects of their wider social environments and the consequences of these for the ways in which their lives unfold. An appreciation of the environmental influences on health behaviour may avoid stereotyping poor health behaviour as the mere failings of individuals and help the recognition that health-supporting environments encourage positive health behaviour.

Moving beyond the level of individual behaviour involves targeting communities with high levels of deprivation and associated ill-health. Government strategy is beginning to move in this direction and to recognise that health inequalities cannot be tackled by the NHS alone (Chapter 11). Local Strategic Partnerships are expected to develop between health and local government, schools, and social services in order to turn national targets into local action. This policy involves not only initiatives to improve the social environments in which people live (e.g. improved local recreational facilities, local facilities to help people stop smoking), but also stresses the actions that individuals can take to improve their own lives (e.g. by actually taking advantage of local recreational facilities and enrolling on smoking cessation programmes). In terms of the 'layers of influence model' (Fig. 3.2), pathways from the 'outside in' (the social environment influencing the individual) are stressed alongside pathways from the 'inside out' (the individual influencing their personal social environment). Nurses and other health care providers will have a role to play in implementing such national, regional and local policies to tackle health inequalities. In particular, the work of primary health services (PHS) has been broadened considerably to include not only service delivery (i.e. the effective diagnosis and treatment of individuals and their specific health problems), but also improving the general health of the wider local population.

Strategies that aim to reduce socio-economic health inequalities work alongside strategies that aim to improve the overall health of the population. Paradoxically, the latter may exacerbate socio-economic health inequalities. Take smoking as an example: health promotion strategies which focus on individual health behaviours are typically taken up more readily by those with better personal and local resources, i.e. those in higher socio-economic groups. Thus even though there has been an overall reduction in cigarette smoking in Britain, as we saw earlier there has been a widening socio-economic gap in smoking (Shaw & Smith 2001). Similarly, the 'better-off' may take advantage of improvements in local areas, such as renovated housing and better shops selling fresh food produce. For these reasons, health improvement initiatives need to be targeted at specifically identified vulnerable groups. At the time of writing (late 2002), it is too early to present a coherent national picture of the kinds of actions that will be taken in primary care to tackle health inequalities but a range of initiatives are underway. These involve partnerships between Primary Care teams and other agencies and include Healthy Living Programmes, Healthy Schools and Healthy Workplace Initiatives (DoH 2002). However, health inequalities cannot be adequately addressed simply at the level of individuals and communities in isolation from other aspects of society. The only long-term solutions to reducing health inequalities are policies that help to reduce economic inequalities and deprivation in the wider society.

Summary

The chapter has reviewed the current evidence on socio-economic inequalities in health and examined explanations for these. Although its focus has been upon Britain, most of the issues raised are also relevant to other advanced industrial societies. The long history of health inequalities underscores their resilience, while more recent research shows that they are increasing. There is now a general acceptance in research and policy circles that health inequalities are socially caused, and that the major determinant is socio-economic inequality within society. Research on the biological, temporal and psychosocial pathways between socio-economic status and health are beginning to provide a better understanding of the relationships between socio-economic inequalities and health inequalities. This poses a challenge to researchers, but also to nurses and other health care providers as they are increasingly expected to take a lead role in reducing health inequalities.

References

Acheson Report (1998) *Independent Inquiry into Inequalities in Health.* The Stationery Office, London.

Arblaster, L. & Hastings, A. (2000) Socio-economic inequality: beyond the inverse care law. In: *Contemporary Primary Care* (ed. P. Tovey). Open University Press, Buckingham.

Barker, D.J.P. (1995) Fetal origins of coronary heart disease. *British Medical Journal,* **311**, 171–174.

Blane, D. (1998) Making sense of socio-economic health inequalities. In: *Sociological Perspectives on Health, Illness and Health Care* (eds D. Field & S. Taylor). Blackwell Science, Oxford.

Blane, D. (1999) The life course, the social gradient, and health. In: *Social Determinants of Health* (eds M. Marmot & R.G. Wilkinson). Oxford University Press, Oxford.

Blane, D. & Drever, F. (1998) Inequality among men in standardised years of potential life lost, 1970–93. *British Medical Journal,* **317**, 255–8.

Blaxter, M. (1990) *Health and Lifestyles.* Tavistock/Routledge, London.

Blaxter, M. (2000) Rethinking social structure and health. In: *Health, Medicine and Society* (eds S. Williams, J. Gabe & M. Calnan). Routledge, London.

Bunting, J. (1997) Morbidity and health-related behaviours of adults – a review. In: *Health*

Inequalities. Decennial Supplement (eds F. Drever & M. Whitehead). Stationery Office, London.

Bury, M. (1997) *Health and Illness in a Changing Society.* Routledge, London.

Coburn, D. (2000) Income inequality, social cohesion and the health status of populations: the role of neo-liberalism. *Social Science and Medicine,* **51**, 135–146.

Davey Smith, G. (1996) Income inequality and mortality: why are they related? *British Medical Journal,* **312**, 988–92.

Davey Smith, G., Dorling, D. & Shaw, M. (eds) (2001) *Poverty, Inequality and Health in Britain 1800–2000: A Reader.* The Policy Press, Bristol.

DoH (2001) *Tackling Health Inequalities. Consultation plan for delivery.* The Stationery Office, London.

DoH (2002) *Health and Neighbourhood Renewal.* The Stationery Office, London.

Drever, F., Fisher, K., Brown, J. & Clark, J (2000) *Social Inequalities. 2000 Edition.* The Stationery Office, London.

Goddard, M. & Smith, P. (2001) Equity of access to health care services: theory and evidence from the UK. *Social Science and Medicine,* **53**, 1149–62.

Graham, H. (2000) Socio-economic change and inequalities in men and women's health in the UK. In: *Gender Inequalities in Health* (eds E. Annandale & K. Hunt). Open University Press, Buckingham.

Lynch, J.W., Davey Smith, G., Kaplan, G. & House, S.J. (2000) Income inequality and mortality: importance to health of individual income, psychosocial environment, or material conditions. *British Medical Journal,* **320**, 1200–1204.

ONS (2001) *Living in Britain.* The Stationery Office, London.

Popay, J., Williams, G., Thomas, C., & Gatrell, T. (1998) Theorising inequalities in health: the place of lay knowledge. *Sociology of Health and Illness,* **20**, 619–44.

Popay, J. & Groves, K. (2000) 'Narrative' in research on gender inequalities in health. In: *Gender Inequalities in Health* (eds E. Annandale & K. Hunt). Open University Press, Buckingham.

Power, C., Bartley, M., Davey Smith, G., & Blane, D. (1996) Transmission of social and biological risk across the lifecourse. In: *Health and Social Organisation* (eds D. Blane, R. Brunner & R. Wilkinson). Routledge, London.

Shaw, M., Dorling, D., Gordon, D. & Davey Smith, G. (1999) *The Widening Gap. Health Inequalities and Policy in Britain.* The Policy Press, Bristol.

Shaw, R. & Smith, P. (2001) Allocating health care resources to reduce health inequalities. *Health Care UK,* **Spring**, 7–13.

Townsend, P., Davidson, N. & Whitehead, M. (1988) *Inequalities in Health.* Penguin, London.

Tudor Hart, J. (1971) The Inverse Care Law. *Lancet,* **I**, 405–412.

Wadsworth, M. (1999) Early Life. In: *Social Determinants of Health* (eds M. Marmot & R.G. Wilkinson). Oxford, Oxford University Press.

Wilkinson, R. (1996) *Unhealthy Societies. The Afflictions of Inequality.* Routledge, London.

Wilkinson, R. (2000) *Mind the Gap. Hierarchies, Health and Human Evolution.* Weidenfeld & Nicholson, London.

Further reading

Graham, H. (ed.) (2000) *Understanding Health Inequalities.* Open University Press, Buckingham.

Marmot, M. & Wilkinson, R.G. (eds) (1999) *Social Determinants of Health.* Oxford University Press, Oxford.

Chapter 4
Ethnicity, Race and Variations in Health

Ethnicity and 'race' are important in the study of health and health care because these social divisions play a significant part in shaping the patterns of health and illness. Ethnic divisions and inequalities have a significant impact on health services and patients' experience of them although they must be seen alongside the impact of other social divisions such as social class. Concepts of 'race' and ethnicity are not just terms to be applied to minority groups supposedly at the margins of society. Everyone has a 'racial' and an ethnic identity. For instance the 'racial' or ethnic group the nurse belongs to, or is *perceived* to belong to by the patient, might carry a particular set of meanings for the patient, or affect the nursing relationship in various ways. This chapter will:

- Define concepts of 'race' and ethnicity
- Provide an overview of the main minority ethnic groups in the UK
- Examine ethnic variations in health
- Review explanations for ethnic variations in health
- Summarise the implications for health services and health care

Race and Ethnicity

Race

Historically, the term 'race' was used to draw distinctions between different groups of human beings that were based on *presumed* physical differences. Actual physical or biological differences are relatively superficial, but race has become a highly important *social* distinction because of powerful beliefs or myths about the intrinsic nature of different 'races', such as intelligence or skills. Racial characteristics cannot be used to explain differences between people but, in everyday life, racial stereotyping leads to assumptions being made about people's behaviour. For people with racist prejudices, the difference between 'black' and 'white' skin signifies deeper differences that derive from beliefs about differences in behaviour and, possibly, the innate superiority of one 'race' over another.

Ethnicity and ethnic relations

Prejudice and discrimination can also arise in relations between ethnic groups. While ethnicity and race are overlapping social categories, ethnicity refers to the ways that social groups can be distinguished from one another according to their cultures and ways of life. The United Kingdom has strong elements of a shared culture marked, for instance, by the use of English as a common language. However, the UK also contains a number of indigenous cultures and two official languages (English and Welsh). There are marked cultural differences, as well as a shared British identity, among English, Irish, Scottish and Welsh groups. In addition there are minority ethnic groups such as the Jewish community, various European minorities (for instance Italian and Polish communities), and African, African Caribbean and Asian minority communities. Included in the latter are people who are migrants, or who are the descendants of migrants, from Bangladesh, Pakistan and India – for instance Sikhs from northern India, or Gujerati-speaking people from western India. However, an ethnic group cannot be summed up simply as a community with a single, distinctive culture. There are three main reasons for this.

First, 'culture' is itself a complex and constantly changing mix of attitudes and beliefs, uses of language and accent, and cultural practices relating to dress, food, marriage, birth, health, illness and death. Cultures are never static – for instance, the outlook and attitudes of Bengali teenagers in East London today are very different from those of their migrant parents or grandparents. There is no single Bengali or Bangladeshi identity in Britain, and this point can be extended to all other ethnic communities.

Second, ethnicity is more than culture. Ethnic identity includes a people's sense of shared history and origins, and of a common destiny. Thus there can be a political dimension to ethnicity. Some ethnic groups develop political and religious organisations to defend or promote their interests, and in some countries there are ethnic political parties. In some respects belonging to an ethnic group that is highly conscious of its identity and distinctiveness can provide the kind of social solidarity, support and meaning in life that is beneficial for health, as discussed in Chapter 2. In other respects belonging to a minority community in a rapidly changing society can cause tensions. Some individuals are torn between the moral codes and social expectations of their ethnic community or family group and the apparent freedoms of the larger society. This might have negative consequences for health as illustrated, for instance, by above-average rates of mental health problems in some ethnic groups.

Third, ethnicity can also be seen as 'more than culture' in the sense that it represents a set of structural influences affecting the standard of living and material circumstances in which individuals and groups live (Nazroo 2001). In some ways this reflects the importance of the social class positions of people in minority communities and the social and economic context in which they exist. Some ethnic minorities (such as the Bangladeshi community) include disproportionately high numbers of economically or socially disadvantaged people, while others (such as the Indian community) do not. However, the structural aspects of ethnicity represent more than the indirect impact of the class structure. Different minority communities are concentrated in different neighbourhoods or urban areas, and the environmental effects of living in each of these locations could explain some of the ethnic variations in health and illness rates that have been observed (Nazroo 2001).

Racial and ethnic divisions and social inequalities in contemporary Britain occur because different ethnic groups have different social status, power and economic resources. Different concepts of *minority* status are a key to understanding this point. Some ethnic groups, for example the Jewish or Italian communities in Britain, might be in a minority, but are not particularly disadvantaged or discriminated against. In these cases, the majority generally accepts the right of the minority to maintain a degree of cultural difference. However, the values and beliefs of some ethnic minority communities are in conflict with dominant values which may foster hostility, discrimination and intolerance on both sides. The status or identity of a minority ethnic community is not static but may change over time so that it is no longer labelled an 'immigrant' minority.

Discrimination against members of minority ethnic groups takes different forms. A basic distinction is between *direct* 'racial' or ethnic discrimination and *indirect* or institutional discrimination. Direct discrimination occurs when individuals act on their prejudices or beliefs to affect the welfare or opportunities of others. Indirect discrimination refers to a pattern of discrimination that arises at the organisational level. Disadvantage to a particular 'racial' or ethnic group may stem from the established working practices and culture of an organisation, even though these may be unintended and unrecognised. It has been argued that problems of institutional or indirect racism can be found in all the major institutions of contemporary British society, including the National Health Service. These can be difficult to deal with because this form of discrimination exists when the organisation treats everyone alike and *appears* to be fair. Paradoxically, treating everyone alike and 'not wanting to discriminate' can lead to a failure to recognise entrenched problems of racial inequality. In preventive health care, for example, a local strategy on cervical screening that treated all women alike might miss important differences in the values and attitudes of different ethnic communities. Also, some health problems are more common in minority ethnic communities than in the majority population, while others are less common. These differences need to be recognised if the NHS is to provide an equal service to all sections of our culturally and ethnically diverse society.

Minority ethnic communities in Britain

A picture of the composition of ethnic communities in Britain can be gained from looking at the UK population census, which included a question about 'ethnic' identity for the first time in 1991. In the 2001 census nearly 8% of the UK's population defined themselves as members of minority ethnic groups compared to 6% in 1991. Most of these belonged to communities with origins in Caribbean and African countries (2.2%) or the Indian subcontinent (3.4%). There are also significant ethnic minorities with roots in Europe (e.g. the Irish community) and in other parts of the world. The minority ethnic population increased from 3 million in 1991 to 4.6 million in 2001. Minority ethnic groups in contemporary Britain have a younger age structure, with less than 5% of people over the age of 65 compared with about 17% in the population as a whole (Scott *et al.* 2001). They also have higher birth rates than the national average. These demographic characteristics affect both their demand

Social Patterns in Health and Disease

for and use of health services. A summary of the main minority ethnic groups can be seen in Table 4.1. Table 4.2 shows the percentage of each ethnic group born in the UK.

While the census picture is of the whole population it gives both a misleading and a partial view of Britain's minority communities. The key point here is that the concept of ethnicity can be defined in different ways (Chapter 1). The main categories used in the 1991 and 2001 censuses are not ethnic groups in the sense defined above. The census refers to 'ethnic groups', but the official categories that householders were asked to choose between, when completing the census, are a mixture of *racial* categories (black or white) and *nationalities* or geographical regions (African, Bangladeshi, Chinese, Indian, Pakistani). 'Indian', for example, is not an ethnic group because the country India is populated by a host of different ethnic communities. Another problem with census definitions of 'race' and ethnicity is that the 'white' category is not subdivided into ethnic or national sub-groups. This

Table 4.1   Population of Great Britain by ethnic group and age, 2000-01 (%). Crown copyright.

Ethnic groups	Under 16	16–34	35–64	65+	All ages (millions)
White	20	25	39	16	53.0
Black Caribbean	23	27	40	10	0.5
Black African	33	35	30	2	0.4
Other Black groups	52	29	17	2	0.3
Indian	23	31	38	8	1.0
Pakistani	36	36	24	4	0.7
Bangladeshi	39	36	21	4	0.3
Chinese	19	38	38	5	0.1
All other minority groups	30	34	33	3	0.8
All ethnic groups	20	26	39	15	57.1

Source   Social Trends No. 32, Office for National Statistics (2002). Adapted from Table 1.4.

Table 4.2   Ethnic groups in the UK, and percentages born in the UK, 1995. Crown copyright.

Ethnic group	% of total population	% Born in the UK
White	94.5	95.8
Black Caribbean	0.9	53.7
Black African	0.4	36.4
Other Black groups	0.3	84.4
Indian	1.5	43.0
Pakistani	0.9	50.5
Bangladeshi	0.3	36.7
Chinese	0.3	28.4
All other minority groups	0.9	44.9

Source   Black and Minority Ethnic Groups in England: the Second Health and Lifestyles Survey, Health Education Authority (2000). Adapted from Figure 1.

implies that being white is an unproblematic, 'non-ethnic' majority status. Being 'ethnic', on the other hand, seems to be a property of being black or Asian, and in a minority.

As 'official' or census definitions of ethnicity are somewhat misleading, it is often more helpful to recognise the ethnic differences between communities that are acknowledged by the communities themselves, as well by outsiders. Table 4.3 identifies the largest minority ethnic groups in contemporary Britain based upon religious, cultural, community and language differences that mark out ethnic identity. It is important to stress that it is not a comprehensive list. Important groups, such as white European minority communities other than the Irish, are missing. There is, to date, little substantial research on health and illness in these communities. The health experiences of 'new' or recent migrants who have arrived as refugees or asylum seekers (e.g. Albanians) or of other small minority communities (e.g. Somalis) are also little researched.

Table 4.3 The largest minority ethnic groups in the UK.

Irish – forming the UK's single largest ethnic minority of about a million people, this community comprises people who migrated to settle in the UK from the Republic of Ireland and Northern Ireland, and their descendants.

African Caribbeans – those who have migrated from countries in the Caribbean, and their descendants.

Black Africans – people who migrated from African countries (chiefly in West Africa) and their descendants.

Indian Sikhs – people who have migrated from the northern Indian state of Punjab, and their descendants, who speak Punjabi and follow the Sikh religion.

Indian Gujeratis – mainly people who migrated from the western Indian state of Gujerat, and their descendants, who speak Gujerati and who are mainly either Hindus or Muslims.

Pakistani Muslims – almost all Pakistanis (and Bangladeshis) follow the religion of Islam. This community includes people and their descendants from various parts of Pakistan, including the northern state of Mirpur and the Pakistani region of Punjab (bordering on Indian Punjab).

Bangladeshi Muslims – migrants and their descendants from coastal areas and from Sylhet, an inland area of Bangladesh.

'African' Asians – migrants or refugees and their descendants, who had been living in various East African countries (e.g. Kenya, Uganda, Tanzania) before settling in the UK. This is a mixed group, in terms of religion and languages, and includes Sikhs, Hindus and Muslims.

Health and illness in minority ethnic communities

The United Kingdom's ethnic diversity in terms of culture, standards of living and experience of 'racial' disadvantage is reflected in ethnic diversity in patterns of health and illness. There is no simple 'racial' divide in health, with the white majority being in a uniformly better off position in respect of rates of illness or mortality. Nor do all black and Asian people share similar rates of illness or experience of health services. However, some clear patterns of health and illness in minority ethnic communities, compared with the white majority, have been identified in recent research. These can be summarised as follows:

- Risks of poorer health and higher death rates are greater in most, but not all, ethnic minority communities
- Indian and African Asian communities have similar, and in some respects better, levels of health compared to the white majority
- most ethnic minorities have *lower* rates of disease and mortality than the white population with regard to respiratory problems, lung and breast cancer
- in Asian communities, the rates for diabetes and coronary heart disease are significantly higher than in the white majority
- in the African Caribbean community the rates for hypertension, stroke and diabetes are significantly higher than in the white majority

These patterns underline the point that the relationship between ethnicity and health is a complex and changing one. Table 4.4 shows the prevalence of common conditions related to the circulatory system by ethnic group. These will be considered, as will mental illness, and two conditions found primarily within ethnic minority communities, tuberculosis and sickle cell disorders.

Table 4.4　Prevalence of selected illnesses by ethnic group (percentages*).

	African Caribbean	Indian	Pakistani	Bangladeshi	England (1994)
Men					
High blood pressure	17	12	9	11	15
Diabetes	9	7	10	12	3
Stroke	2	2	1	3	2
Angina	3	3	2	8	**
Heart attack	3	2	4	4	4
N	*929*	*1497*	*1752*	*1859*	
Women					
High blood pressure	30	15	12	11	18
Diabetes	9	5	8	11	2
Stroke	1	1	1	0.4	2
Angina	3	2	1	5	**
Heart attack	1	1	1	1	2
N	*1043*	*1492*	*1729*	*1682*	

*Percentages have been rounded
** Angina and heart attack were combined in the data for England
Source　Black and Ethnic Minority Groups in England: the Second Health and Lifestyles Survey, Health Education Authority (2000). Adapted from Figure 4.1.

Heart disease

Balarajan (1995) and Whitehead *et al.* (1988) draw attention to the problem of excess deaths from coronary heart disease (CHD) among men and women in South Asian communities. Taken as a whole, people who have migrated from the Indian subcontinent to the UK are more than half as likely again to die of CHD than people in the majority population. Balarajan found the proportion of excess CHD deaths (above the average in England and Wales) to be 73% among Bangladeshis, 61% among Pakistanis, and 53% among Indians (1995). These death rates exceed the rate for England and Wales that is already high by international standards.

More recently a large-scale survey of the UK's ethnic groups (Modood *et al.* 1997) has qualified this picture. Reporting on this research, Nazroo points out that while risk of contracting heart disease appears to be significantly higher among South Asians, compared to the white majority, 'this greater risk applied only to the Pakistani/Bangladeshi group' (Nazroo 1997). In this survey, Indian and African Asian respondents were found to have the same risk of heart disease as whites. Another survey, for the Health Education Authority (2000), also found significant differences *between* these minority ethnic communities in the proportions of people who had been told that they had angina, or had suffered heart attacks. The Bangladeshi group emerged in this survey as a community experiencing 'strikingly worse levels of general health, including ... heart disease' (HEA 2000). Nazroo (1997) concludes that, just as there is a strong relationship between social class and CHD in the majority population, class differences also explain many 'ethnic' differences in heart disease. According to him, once socio-economic status is taken into account the risk of diagnosed heart disease as compared to whites drops for all South Asian communities, and falls to insignificant levels for the Pakistani/ Bangladeshi group.

Thus, as far as heart disease is concerned, inequalities in the incomes, material resources and occupations of people in the different minorities are of key importance in understanding the observed variations. This conclusion is confirmed by analysis of risk of CHD *within* ethnic groups, which shows a marked class gradient in each of the main South Asian communities in the UK and in different parts of India (Nazroo 1997).

Hypertension and stroke

Hypertension (high blood pressure) is a significant risk factor in causing stroke, or haemorrhage in the brain. Rates of hypertension vary significantly across ethnic groups and between men and women, although caution is necessary in interpreting the epidemiological evidence. This is because raised blood pressure may not be noticed until the patient is examined or treated for something else. Research on hypertension and the occurrence of strokes in different ethnic groups has produced consistent findings. Balarajan (1995), for instance, points to an excess of deaths from stroke among older African Caribbeans (aged 65–74) that is 50% higher than the norm in England and Wales. He also shows that deaths from stroke are even higher in the Bangladeshi community (twice the England and Wales rate), significantly above in the Indian community, and slightly above the rate in the Pakistani community.

Although the risk of death from stroke is high in some Asian communities, the danger of hypertension has frequently been referred to in health research as an African Caribbean problem. For example, Balarajan (2001) points out that 'African Caribbeans around the globe are known to suffer disproportionately from hypertensive disease and stroke.' International studies of hypertension in African American and Caribbean populations seemed to confirm a 'racial' difference, with black communities experiencing a significantly higher rate of hypertension than whites in all age groups. Medical research therefore began to conclude that genetic factors were strongly linked to a predisposition towards hypertension in all people of black African descent. However more recent research (McKeigue 2001), including careful comparison of rural and urban communities in Africa, has shown that rates of hypertension and stroke are not uniformly high in all black communities. Where they are particularly high, notably in relatively disadvantaged black communities in the USA, they seem to be closely associated with adverse environmental factors. McKeigue suggests that poverty, unhealthy high-calorie diets and obesity play a key role in causing significantly higher rates of these health problems.

Diabetes

A significantly high rate of diabetes was observed in black and South Asian minority ethnic communities through earlier research on immigrants to the UK (e.g. Marmot *et al*. 1984). More recent studies, which include both the immigrant generation and their UK-born descendants (Nazroo 1997, HEA 2000), have confirmed – as with hypertension and stroke – that the incidence of diabetes in most African Caribbean and Asian communities has remained at a significantly higher level in the succeeding, UK-born generations. Nazroo (1997), reporting data from the Fourth National Survey (see Modood *et al*. 1997) shows that Pakistani and Bangladeshi communities experience over five times the rate of diabetes found in the white population (8.9% compared to 1.7%, standardised for age and gender). The rates of diabetes in the African Caribbean group were found to be over three times higher (5.3%), and in the Indian and African Asian communities to be just under three times higher (4.7%), than in the white population. The Chinese group had the lowest rate among the minorities surveyed (3.0%), although this is still appreciably higher than in the white majority.

Nazroo (1997) shows that these ethnic differences in rates of diabetes remain significant even when socio-economic status is controlled for. In other words, diabetes rates are still significantly higher in middle-class or better-off sections of minority communities, as well as in poorer or less advantaged sections, when equivalent comparisons are made with the white majority. For this reason, some researchers have suggested that genetic factors could play an important part in causing relatively high rates of diabetes in black and Asian groups (Chandola 2001). However, even in the case of diabetes it is not entirely clear how genetic differences alone could account for increased susceptibility to insulin intolerance and diabetes in these groups. Environmental and dietary factors also play an important part in explaining a marked global rise in diabetes in recent years. Complex interactions between genetic inheritance, changing diets and other environmental changes are most likely to explain the observed ethnic differences in this serious and growing health problem.

Tuberculosis

The rising incidence of this disease in the UK and the USA is a cause for concern. The appearance of resistant strains means that tuberculosis (TB) cannot be controlled as easily as it was in the past. In the UK disproportionate emphasis was initially placed on a higher rate of TB in migrants' home countries to explain the higher rate in minority ethnic communities. In fact, the incidence of TB was found to be low in some countries of origin, notably the Caribbean states (Donovan 1984). Further, a growing proportion of black and Asian British people have been born in the UK (Table 4.2). Most of those who contract TB do so as a result of living conditions in the UK, rather than as a result of contact with people in other countries. More recently, however, there does seem to have been a rise in the rate of TB as a result of contact between UK citizens and people living in poorer countries where rates of TB are very high. In 2002, the rate in London was four times higher than the European average and in certain areas, the incidence of TB was equivalent to the levels for countries such as China, Russia and Brazil. However, it is important to stress that the recent rise of TB in London and other major British cities reflects a complex combination of contributory factors, including poverty and low standards of accommodation as well as foreign travel and population movement. Some minority ethnic communities, particularly the Pakistani and Bangladeshi minorities, experience a disproportionate amount of social disadvantage and researchers suggest that ethnic differences in rates of TB are largely a result of poverty, poor diet and housing and unemployment (Bhopal 2001).

Sickle cell disorders

The example of tuberculosis illustrates the important link between illness and living conditions (Chapter 3). However, there are several kinds of disease in which this link is unimportant and which can only be explained by genetic differences between ethnic groups. Inherited conditions such as sickle cell disorders are not entirely unknown in the majority population but they are much more closely associated with specific minority communities.

Sickle cell disorders are inherited disorders of haemoglobin in the red blood cells. They include '*sickle cell anaemia* (usually the more severe type), *haemoglobin SC disease* (usually milder) and sickle cell beta *thalassaemia* (of which there is both a severe and a mild form)' (Anionwu 1993). As many as one in four West African adults and one in ten adults from the Caribbean carry the sickle cell trait. Thalassaemia is carried by one in seven Cypriot adults (and is also found in other eastern Mediterranean populations), and between one in 15 to 30 Chinese adults. It is also found in other Asian populations, and among one in 50 African Caribbean adults. Carriers do not suffer from the painful and dangerous effects of these blood disorders, even in a mild form. Its presence as a trait has been associated with resistance to malaria – hence its geographical distribution in world regions where malaria is, or was, common. When both parents are carriers, there is a one in four chance that their children will experience illness as a result of a sickle cell disorder.

Greater awareness of sickle cell disorders is needed because, as Anionwu (1993) and others have pointed out, the record of the NHS in providing help and information, genetic counselling and treatment has been patchy and inadequate in this area.

Mental illness

Whether minority ethnic groups have poorer mental health than the majority population is a question surrounded by controversy. This is because of the difficulties of obtaining reliable statistics of its prevalence and because mental illness itself is difficult to define (Chapter 8). Responses to illness are affected to some degree by cultural values and social stereotypes and this is particularly the case with mental illness. Psychiatric diagnoses have a record of unreliability, and there is concern about the impact of this on black and Asian patients (Sashidharan & Francis 1993). It seems that the prevalence of some forms of mental illness in minority communities might have been over-estimated (perhaps greatly) by medical research.

There is strong evidence (summarised by Nazroo & King 2002) that African Caribbean and African people are much more likely than whites to be admitted to hospital with a first diagnosis of schizophrenia or other psychotic illnesses. Younger men experience particularly high rates of hospitalisation. Research has suggested that cultural misunderstandings have been influencing psychiatrists' and other health practitioners' perceptions of their needs. Earlier studies also showed that black patients were likely to be dealt with more coercively than white patients with the same symptoms of mental illness (Littlewood & Lipsedge 1989). While it has been argued that the psychological impact of racism could be an important factor explaining mental illness between minority ethnic groups, it cannot explain variations in rates of mental illness within them.

There are concerns that some mental health problems among minority ethnic groups and the distress they cause might be being missed by researchers and by health service providers. One of the main weaknesses of early research on ethnic variations in mental illness was that much of it was based on surveys of treatment or admission to hospital. This made interpretation of results difficult, as a wide variety of reasons other than mental illness itself could explain why higher numbers of people from certain ethnic groups were receiving institutional treatment. For example, the impression of a very high incidence of schizophrenia in the black community was created by a series of epidemiological studies that were based on hospital admission rates (Littlewood & Lipsedge 1989; Sashidharan & Francis 1993). These showed rates of hospital admission of African Caribbean people for schizophrenia that were between 3 and 17 times higher than in the majority population. Of all patients admitted to mental hospitals surveyed in these studies, between 40–50% of African Caribbean patients were diagnosed as schizophrenic while fewer than one in seven white British patients received this diagnosis.

Three large sample surveys (Modood *et al.* 1997; Nazroo 1997, Sproston & Nazroo 2002) provide more reliable findings on the prevalence of mental health problems in different ethnic groups using evidence based on mental illness rates in the community, rather than on treatment or hospitalisation rates. In terms of a set of common mental disorders such as anxiety, low mood and irritability, the most recent survey (Sproston & Nazroo 2002) found relatively minor differences between ethnic groups (including the white majority). No ethnic group stood out as being particularly susceptible to common mental disorders, although there are differences between the experience of men and women in various ethnic groups. For example, Irish men and Pakistani women were found to have significantly higher rates of common mental disorders as compared to their counterparts in the majority community.

When specific disorders such as anxiety and depression were analysed separately, some ethnic differences emerged. Nazroo (1997) reports a significantly higher rate of depression in the African Caribbean community (more than 40% above that found in the white majority). Reported symptoms of anxiety were particularly low in the Indian community. The Bangladeshi community, the most economically disadvantaged, was found in the Department of Health survey (Sproston & Nazroo 2002) to experience the lowest rates of a range of common mental disorders. These results suggest that there is no clear link between ethnic group, material disadvantage and common mental disorders. This contrasts with ethnic inequalities in heart disease and the other physical health problems discussed earlier, which do seem to reflect underlying patterns of class inequality and economic disadvantage in minority ethnic groups.

Differences in social support and integration (Chapter 2) seem to mediate the effects of economic disadvantage and racial discrimination in producing ethnic differences in rates of common mental disorders. Sproston and Nazroo (2002) suggest that social support and 'community social capital' can offset the effects of social deprivation, protecting some groups, for example the Bangladeshi community, from a higher rate of mental health problems. African Caribbean communities, although supportive and a source of identity and help, are more likely to include socially isolated people living on their own than would be the case in most South Asian communities (Blakemore & Boneham 1994). This might have increased African Caribbean people's vulnerability to the psychological effects of social disadvantage.

Explaining ethnic variation in health and illness

The previous section has indicated a number of explanations for ethnic differences in health and suggested that there is no single explanation for them.

Genetic explanations

These seem to have limited explanatory power because the incidence of most of the health conditions discussed seemed to vary as much *within* ethnic groups as between them. If genetic factors mainly determined rates of disease, there would no significant differences in disease rates within groups. The main exception was diabetes, although environmental factors, particularly changes in diet, seem to be strongly implicated in both a general rise in rates of diabetes and increases in the African Caribbean community. Inherited blood disorders such as sickle cell disorders in certain minority communities, clearly do have a genetic cause and are only very rarely found in the majority white population.

Cultural explanations

Cultural and lifestyle factors such as differences in smoking, diet and taking exercise have been closely associated with differences in health, particularly by governments in their public health and health promotion policies (Chapter 2, Chapter 3). Evidence to support this explanation for ethnic health differences can be found in the significantly lower rates of respiratory disease and lung cancer found in South Asian communities, compared to both the African Caribbean community and the white majority, attributed mainly to the very low rates of smoking among South Asian women (Nazroo 2001), suggesting that some cultural values and social habits have an enhancing impact on health. However, there is little evidence that other cultural or lifestyle differences between ethnic groups are very significant. Reviewing the evidence on unhealthy diets, lack of exercise and resistance to using medical services, Chandola (2001) concludes that it would be incorrect to attribute poorer health in South Asian or black communities to such health-damaging behaviours. These are unlikely to have any more effect in these communities than in the white majority. Also, if cultural factors such as dietary habits are common to an ethnic group, they cannot explain significant differences *within* ethnic groups in rates of serious illness. Focusing on cultural explanations for health inequalities at the expense of other factors can result in 'blaming the victim' for their own poorer health and in downplaying the structural and environmental causes of illness.

Racism and racial disadvantage

This suggests that racial discrimination and disadvantage undermine health in various ways. Racial discrimination can be *indirect* or institutional, subtly affecting people's opportunities in education, employment, housing and other aspects of life that determine standards of living. Thus the health of some minority ethnic groups could be adversely affected because rates of illness are closely connected to inequalities in standard of living. The *direct*, personal, impact of racism could have a wide range of psychological effects, including anxiety and other mental health problems, and physical effects of stress such as high blood pressure.

The impact on health of racism seems to vary. If discrimination affects everyone perceived to be 'black' or 'Asian' in approximately the same ways and to the same degree, we would expect to see approximately the same outcomes across the minority groups. But as Chandola (2001) reminds us, there are significant differences in both illness and death rates between Indian men on one hand, and Bangladeshi and Pakistani men on the other. Significant differences in standard of living *within* ethnic groups suggest that for various reasons, including social class position, some sections within minority ethnic communities can protect themselves better against the effects of racial discrimination on their health. The protective effect of belonging to an ethnic group is not solely dependent on economic and social position. Low rates of anxiety in the Indian community and of common mental disorders in the Bangladeshi community suggest that strong social support could be another factor mitigating the effects of racism on mental health.

Migration and social selection

The migrant background of black, Asian, Irish and other minority communities in the UK provides another set of explanations for ethnic variations in health. Migration can be seen as having both positive and negative effects. First, as Marmot *et al.* (1984) pointed out in an early study of death rates among migrants to the UK, migrants are a self-selected group. Their health tends to be better than that of the populations from which they have come and they bring a certain advantage in health and life expectancy with them. This seems to be confirmed by a number of studies of migrant death rates. In the 1950s and 1960s, mortality rates among men in social classes IV and V of these groups were *lower* than among their white counterparts in the same social classes and age groups (Whitehead *et al.* 1988). Among women, deaths from breast cancer were less than half the rate among migrants from the Indian subcontinent, compared with the average in Britain, and were fewer in all the minority groups (Balarajan 1995). However, it is possible for the ethnic minority's *death* rate to be lower than average and for their rates of *illness*, at least for certain diseases, to be higher than the norm. One of the criticisms of earlier studies of ethnicity and health is that too much emphasis was put upon mortality statistics and not enough on illness rates.

As the migrant generations have aged, they have experienced relatively high rates of heart disease, hypertension, diabetes and other health problems. Some negative aspects of migration, such as loss of support, stress and psychological problems of adjustment, may have played a part in increasing these health problems. However, when the health of migrant Asian and black people is compared with non-migrants in the same communities, in most cases migrants are found to have better physical and mental health (Nazroo 2001). These findings suggest first, that the shock, stress and disruption of migration cannot have had a very significant effect on migrants' health, and cannot be used to explain ethnic variations in illness rates. It also appears that the 'health advantage' of the migrant generation has not been transmitted in any significant way to the second and third generations of minority ethnic groups in contemporary Britain.

Socio-economic status differences

Many of what *appear* to be ethnic variations in health and illness can be explained by examining the impact of socio-economic status or social class on the comparisons being made. Of all the explanations considered, this one has perhaps the greatest explanatory power. The comprehensive surveys of ethnic minority health discussed earlier (see Modood *et al.* 1997; Nazroo 1997, Health Education Authority 2000) consistently show that socio-economic status is centrally important when making comparisons between ethnic groups. However, socio-economic status does not explain every variation in health between ethnic groups. As will be recalled, exceptions include the distribution of diabetes, which is significantly higher in minority black and Asian groups irrespective of socio-economic status. Another exception is the low rate of common mental problems in the economically disadvantaged Bangladeshi community.

Explanations based on socio-economic status also have their limitations when comparisons of health *within* ethnic groups, as opposed to *between* ethnic groups, are being made. For example, Chandola (2001) concluded there was little evidence of a class gradient in health within the relatively disadvantaged Pakistani and Bangladeshi communities. In the Indian community, on the other hand, a significant increase in social mobility since the 1980s and a widening social divide have resulted in widening health inequalities. In the African Caribbean community, there seems to be a mixed picture. According to Nazroo (2001), poorer people in the African Caribbean community generally had poorer health, indicating a class gradient, although there were some exceptions, such as a higher rate of mental illness for those in non-manual occupations, compared with manual workers.

Health services and health care

Although medicine and health care have their limitations in terms of reducing mortality and contributing to positive improvements in health (Chapter 2) health services are of central importance in the management and treatment of illnesses. How they perform these functions in minority ethnic communities is therefore important. There seem to be both positive and negative aspects to the experience of health services among minority groups, so it is important to strike a balance between the view that the NHS is a benign, multicultural organisation that treats all ethnic groups equally and the opposite view that it is an inherently racist service dominated by white professionals.

Positive aspects

Unlike social services, the NHS is a well-understood and well-used service among all the minority ethnic communities (Blakemore & Boneham 1994), and there are no significant problems of under-registration or exclusion from health services. This applies to use of hospital services as well as to GP or family doctor services. As with the white majority, almost everyone in black, Asian and other minority ethnic communities is registered with a GP. African Caribbean men are the only group with lower registration rates (96%) than the general population (Nazroo 1997).

Summarising a number of surveys on use of in-patient hospital services, Nazroo (1997) shows that patients from minority ethnic groups are as likely to be admitted to hospital as whites, taking reported illnesses into account. Younger minority patients are less likely to be admitted to hospital than is the norm in the white population but rates of admission among older South Asian and African Caribbean patients are similar to, or greater than, admissions of white patients. Rates of GP consultations are higher in most minority ethnic groups than in the white population. For example, Nazroo's (1997) survey showed that 35% of white respondents had talked to their GP about their health in the past month, compared with 41–50% of Indian, African Caribbean, Bangladeshi and Pakistani respondents. Only African Asians (32%) reported a lower rate of GP consultations. Ethnic minority patients, compared to whites, are also more likely to visit their GPs more than once each month.

Negative aspects

The pattern of use of NHS services may be an indicator of a heavier burden of illness in minority ethnic communities. There is little evidence that patients from these groups 'over-use' health services or facilities, compared to the white population. Where use of health services is more frequent than the national average this seems to reflect medical need. The use of preventative services, e.g. screening for cervical cancer, is lower than the national average among ethnic minority communities and black and Asian patients are significantly less likely than white patients to receive follow-up services, or to be referred promptly to a consultant if they have a serious illness such as heart disease (Nazroo 1997). Many GPs are unwilling to work in socially disadvantaged or inner city areas where most minority ethnic communities live. GP practices used by patients from minority ethnic groups are not as likely to have good facilities as practices in better-off areas. Also, physical access to the doctor's surgery has been found to be more of a problem for ethnic minority patients than for people in the white majority (Balarajan 2001).

A significant number of South Asian patients report communication problems with their GPs, mainly as a result of language differences. These difficulties mainly affect older patients and women, rather than younger patients and men. As many as a half of Bangladeshi and Pakistani women are likely to have difficulty in communicating in English, and these proportions will be even higher among older women in these communities. Although there are now considerable numbers of South Asian GPs working in the NHS, this does not always mean that doctor and patient will be matched in terms of the Asian languages they can speak. There might also be considerable cultural and status differences between Asian patients and Asian doctors.

The existence of language barriers between doctors and patients is not necessarily a criticism of the NHS as factors that lie outside the control of the health service have helped to maintain these barriers (e.g. limited policies on teaching English to adults; cultural and linguistic preferences in different communities). However, communication problems may partly explain why Asian patients visit their GPs more frequently than white patients. If the doctor has not been well-understood in the first consultation, this increases the chances of the patient having to return for further advice and treatment (Sproston & Nazroo 2002). Efforts to improve communication between family doctors and minority ethnic patients have been patchy (Health Education Authority 2000) and have been hindered by the general shortage of GPs.

Although the NHS has an ethnically and racially diverse work force there is evidence of direct and indirect racism, as well as a lack of understanding of the significance of ethnic and cultural differences. Some researchers have found intolerance among medical practitioners and nurses towards ethnic minority patients, for example the study of GPs by Ahmad *et al.* (1991) and Bowler's (1993) study of midwives. Evidence of indirect discrimination can be observed in the failure of the NHS to reach out sufficiently vigorously to the various minority communities. For instance, take-up of some preventive services is low, especially in Asian communities (Balarajan 2001).

Research on hospitals suggests that nurses' understanding of black and Asian patients' dietary, religious and other cultural needs is sometimes poor and haphazard, although it can be improved with appropriate training and information (Karmi 1996; Mares *et al.* 1985). Patients from minority ethnic groups do not expect to be given special treatment, in terms of medical or nursing care. Rather, their concerns are that the specific cultural practices of their community or requirements of their religious beliefs – in short, their ethnic identity – are understood by nurses and other health care staff. It is in this respect that a sociological understanding of the patient's cultural background and identity can be helpful to nurses. All nursing care takes place in a cultural context and represents, in one sense, a cultural exchange between nurse and patient.

The health and illness behaviours of *all* patients and nurses, including those from the majority white population are shaped by their ethnic and cultural identities. Where the ethnic identities of nurse and patient are similar there are likely to be shared understandings between patient and nurse about:

● How symptoms are described and expressed
● How the body should be washed and cared for
● Problems of excretion
● How to talk about treatment choices
● How to deal with relatives and visitors

Where the care relationship involves a cultural or ethnic difference, a shared understanding of these aspects of nursing cannot be taken for granted. There is a strong case, therefore, for maintaining an element of cultural awareness in the education and training of nurses. This is likely to be at least as valuable as training in awareness of racial discrimination.

Summary

Race and ethnicity are socially constructed categories and, although many people believe that there are 'real' or objective differences between racial and ethnic groups, such beliefs are based on myths of racial superiority/inferiority rather than on valid scientific evidence. Rates of mortality and morbidity between and within ethnic groups do not consistently favour the white majority and in some respects health in minority ethnic communities is better than in the majority. No single explanation – genetic, cultural, socio-economic, migration or 'racial' discrimination – can explain the variations in health between ethnic groups. These are best seen as the outcome of a range of interacting causes. When health status is taken into account, black and Asian patients see their GPs more frequently than white patients and are as likely to be admitted to hospital as whites. While access to health services is not generally a problem for ethnic minority groups, there are barriers to effective communication between some groups of ethnic minority patients and health service practitioners, and shortcomings in health services in areas such as follow-up treatment, preventive services and mental health care.

References

Ahmad, W.I.U., Baker, M. & Kernohan, E. (1991) General practitioners' perceptions of Asian and non-Asian patients'. *Family Practice – an International Journal*, **8**, 52–6.

Anionwu, E.N. (1993) Sickle cell and thalassaemia: community experiences and official response. In: *'Race' and Health in Contemporary Britain* (ed. W.I.U. Ahmad). Open University Press, Buckingham.

Balarajan, R. (1995) Ethnicity and variations in the nation's health. *Health Trends*, **27**, 114–19.

Balarajan, R. (2001) Challenges and policy implications of ethnic diversity and health. In: *Health and Ethnicity* (eds H. Macbeth & P. Shetty). Taylor & Francis, London.

Bhopal, R. (2001) Ethnicity and race as epidemiological variables. In: *Health and Ethnicity* (eds H. Macbeth & P. Shetty). Taylor & Francis, London.

Blakemore, K. & Boneham, M. (1994) *Age, Race and Ethnicity – a Comparative Approach*. Open University Press, Buckingham.

Bowler, I. (1993) 'They're not the same as us': Midwives' stereotypes of South Asian descent maternity patients. *Sociology of Health and Illness*, **15**, 157–78.

Chandola, T. (2001) Ethnic and class differences in health in relation to British South Asians: using the new National Statistics Socio-Economic Classification. *Social Science and Medicine*, **52**, 1285–96.

Donovan, J. (1984) Ethnicity and health: a research review. *Social Science and Medicine*, **19**, 633–70.

Harding, S. & Maxwell, R. (1997) Differences in the mortality of migrants. In: *Health Inequalities* (eds F. Drever & M. Whitehead). The Stationery Office, London.

Health Education Authority (2000) *Black and Ethnic Minority Groups in England: the Second Health and Lifestyles Survey*. Health Education Authority, London.

Karmi, G. (1996) *The Ethnic Health Handbook*. Blackwell Science, Oxford.

Law, I. (1996) *Racism, Ethnicity and Social Policy*. Prentice Hall/ Harvester Wheatsheaf, London.

Littlewood, R. & Lipsedge, M. (1989) *Aliens and Alienists: Ethnic Minorities and Psychiatry* 2nd edn. Unwin Hyman, London.

Mares, P., Henley, A. & Baxter, C. (1985) *Health Care in Multiracial Britain*. Health Education Council and National Extension College, London.

Marmot, M.G., Adelstein, A. & Bulusu, L. (1984) Immigrant mortality in England and Wales, 1970–78: causes of death by country of birth. *Studies on Medical and Population Subjects, No. 47*. HMSO, London.

McKeigue, P. (2001) Approaches to investigating the genetic basis of ethnic differences in disease risk. In: *Health and Ethnicity* (eds H. Macbeth & P. Shetty). Taylor & Francis, London.

Modood, T., Berthoud, R., Lakey, J., Nazroo, J., Smith, P., Virdee, S., & Beishon, S. (1997) *Ethnic Minorities in Britain: Diversity and Disadvantage*. Policy Studies Institute, London.

Nazroo, J. (1997) *The Health of Britain's Ethnic Minorities*. Policy Studies Institute, London.

Nazroo, J. (2001) *Ethnicity, Class and Health*. Policy Studies Institute, London.

Nazroo, J. & King, M. (2002) Psychosis – symptoms and estimated rates. In: *Ethnic Minority Psychiatric Rates in the Community (EMPIRIC)* (eds K. Sproston & J. Nazroo). The Stationery Office, Norwich.

Scott, A., Pearce, D. & Goldblatt D. (2001) The sizes and characteristics of the minority ethnic population of Great Britain – latest estimates. *Population Trends*, **105**, 6–16.

Sashidharan, S.P. & Francis, E. (1993) Epidemiology, ethnicity and schizophrenia. In: *'Race' and Health in Contemporary Britain* (ed. W.I.U. Ahmad). Open University Press, Buckingham.

Sproston, K. & Nazroo, J. (eds) (2002) *Ethnic Minority Psychiatric Illness Rates in the Community (EMPIRIC)*. The Stationery Office, Norwich.

Whitehead, M., with Townsend, P. & Davidson, N. (eds) (1988) *Inequalities in Health: the Black Report and the Health Divide*. Penguin, Harmondsworth.

Wilkinson, P., Sayer, J., Koorithottumkal, L., Grundy, C., Marchant, B., Kopelman, P. and Timmis, A. (1996) Comparison of case fatality in south Asian and white patients after acute myocardial infarction: an observational study. *British Medical Journal*, **312**, 1330–33.

Further reading

Ahmed, W.I. (ed.) (2000) *Ethnicity, disability and chronic illness*. Open University Press, Buckingham.

Nazroo, J. (2001) *Ethnicity, Class and Health*. Policy Studies Institute, London.

Chapter 5
Gender Differences in Health

Research on gender differences in health only began in the 1970s. Nevertheless, an established wisdom quickly emerged, summarised in the widely used phrase *'women are sicker, but men die quicker'*. Research evidence suggested that while women tended to have more illness throughout their lives, men died at younger ages. Two explanations have been suggested for these gender differences in health. First, that they are the result of biological differences between the sexes. Second, that they are the result of gender-related attitudes and behaviours. More recent research has led to the recognition that this summary oversimplifies the complex relationships between gender and health in contemporary British society. Among younger people, in particular, gender roles and behaviours are overlapping and the boundaries between them are becoming blurred. The chapter will:

- Present evidence on gender differences in mortality and morbidity
- Discuss the main explanations for gender differences in health
- Consider the importance of recent changes in gender roles and experiences for the health of men and women

Gender patterns in mortality

In contemporary Britain the marked female advantage in life expectancy is accepted as a 'fact of life'. However, this has not always been the case and it may not hold true in the future. Before the late 1880s, it was men who lived longer. Although the absence of statistical data makes it difficult to give an accurate picture of the distant past, Shorter (1982) maintains that in prehistoric times adult men outlived women at almost all ages. Likewise studies of sixteenth, seventeenth and eighteenth century European villages show a male advantage. By the early Victorian period, statistics assembled by national record offices give a much more reliable picture. For 1840 to around 1860 they show an emerging female advantage in life expectancy of between one and two years. However, this did not hold for all ages; at younger ages (between 10 to 35) girls and women were still much more likely to die than boys and men.

The gradual shift away from male to female advantage in life expectancy was related to changes in women's social circumstances. Death from childbirth was quite common in Victorian times although it was not the main cause of death for women; before the mid- to late 1800s they were far more likely to die from 'killer diseases' like tuberculosis (TB), scarlet fever, typhus and typhoid fever. For example, TB accounted for the deaths of around half of all women aged 15 to 25 in the mid-1800s. Although men were afflicted by the same diseases, women's circumstances made them much more vulnerable to illness and death. As Shorter (1982) explains, 'women were more liable than men to die at certain ages because their lives at those ages were much harder than men's, and their resistance to infection was lower.' Grinding work in the fields in rural areas, chronic exhaustion from maintaining the family, anaemia and malnutrition particularly took their toll. Rapid urbanisation and industrialisation freed many women from the health-damaging effects of rural life. The health problems that industrialisation and urbanisation brought in their wake affected men as much as women.

A new historical period began around the late 1800s when women began to outlive men at all ages. Death rates began to fall significantly, and by the early 1900s men and women could now expect to live, on average, into their late 40s and early 50s. By the early 1970s this had risen to the late 60s to mid-70s. Table 5.1 presents trends in life expectancy over the twentieth century and projected trends for the twenty-first century. We can see that women's 'extra years' increased steadily for those born at the start of the twentieth century to peak at 6.3 years for those born in

Table 5.1 Expectation of life at birth. Crown copyright.

Year of birth	Men	Women	Difference (women's extra years)
*Actual, England and Wales**			
1901–1910	48.5	52.4	3.9
1910–12	51.5	55.4	3.9
1920–22	55.6	59.6	4.0
1930–32	58.7	62.9	4.2
1950–52	66.4	71.5	5.1
1960–62	68.1	74.0	5.9
1970–72	69.0	75.3	6.3
1980–82	71.0	77.0	6.0
1990–92	73.4	79.0	5.6
1993–95	74.1	79.4	5.3
Years of life gained			
1980–1995	3.1	2.4	
Projected, UK			
1999	75.1	79.9	4.8
2011	77.4	81.6	4.2
2021	78.6	82.7	4.1
Years of life gained			
1999-2021	3.5	2.8	

Sources R. Fitzpatrick & R. Chandola (2000) *Twentieth-Century British Social Trends* (eds A.H. Halsey & J. Webb); *National Population Projections 1998-based* (2000) Series PP2, No. 2. ONS.
*Similar patterns are found for Scotland and Northern Ireland (not shown here).

1970–72. The female advantage continued throughout the 1980s and 1990s and is projected to continue for those born in the early decades of the twenty-first century. However, Table 5.1 also shows that the magnitude of women's advantage is declining, a point taken up later in the chapter.

This consideration of history shows that gender differences in mortality are by no means fixed: while men had the advantage in the past, it is women who have the advantage today. This suggests that differences in mortality are unlikely to be a simple product of the biological differences between men and women. Rather they are likely to result from the interaction of the different biological vulnerabilities of men and women and the different circumstances of their lives in different historical periods.

Explaining gender differences in mortality

Biology

It has been suggested that men die sooner because they are more biologically vulnerable and, conversely, that women live longer because they are biologically more robust. Support for 'male vulnerability' comes from studies of the male fetus. Kraemer (2000) argues that for men it is 'downhill from conception to birth'. The male foetus is at greater risk of obstetric complications. Premature birth, stillbirth, cerebral palsy, and congenital malformations of the genitalia and limbs are commoner in male infants. Sudden infant death syndrome, although uncommon, is also more likely to affect boys than girls (ONS 2002). Moreover, at the time of birth boys are on average developmentally some four to six weeks behind girls. The chance of surviving the first year of life is also lower for boys. This suggests that females may be born with a biological advantage.

Further support for 'female robustness' comes from studies of health in later life. For example, coronary heart disease (CHD) is a leading cause of death for both men and women, but it typically affects women at older ages. This later onset may be due to the protective effect of high levels of the female sex-hormone oestrogen. Women's risk of heart disease increases in later life due to the post-menopausal drop in oestrogen levels (Pollard 1999).

The biological body does not exist in isolation, but develops in interaction with the social environment. Any female biological advantage in the first weeks of life can be quickly over-ridden by social preferences for baby boys that confer health advantages such as more food and closer attention to health problems. This is especially notable in some developing countries. Similarly, while oestrogen may protect women from CHD, the secretion of oestrogen by the ovaries is itself influenced by the social environment, particularly the kinds of lifestyles that women lead. Cigarette smoking, which in itself is a risk factor for CHD, appears to reduce women's secretion of oestrogen (and is also associated with an early menopause). Likewise, stress is thought to adversely affect ovarian function.

A final example of how biology is embedded in social experience is the propensity for men to engage in activities that carry a high risk of serious injury or death, such as dangerous sports or physical fighting. This may be associated with high levels of androgen testosterone. However it is also important to recognise that, in most western countries, competition, physical aggression, and risky behaviours are often more actively encouraged among boys and men than among girls and women. Moreover, increases in levels of testosterone may be further stimulated by the anticipation of competition and risk that such encouragement brings (Courtenay 2002). This suggests that far from operating in isolation, it is the *interaction* of biological and social factors that is important.

Social factors

Gender is an important social division between people in modern patriarchal societies such as Britain. Patriarchy is a system of male dominance which advantages men and disadvantages women and traditionally operates by creating a strong gender divide, attributing certain 'natural' biological and psychological characteristics to men and others to women. For example, women are physically weak, men are physically strong; women are naturally caring, men are naturally aggressive; men are competitive, women are co-operative/supportive. These characteristics are often drawn together under the umbrella terms of 'femininity' and 'masculinity'. While feminists have strongly challenged female gender role expectations for decades, and the new discipline of men's studies is now questioning male gender role expectations, the concept of gender roles has had a very strong influence upon explanations of the health and health behaviours of males and females (Annandale 1998).

Gender roles and health behaviours

The conventional wisdom is that the gender roles and behaviours associated with being a man or being a woman in contemporary western society predispose men to early death and, conversely, prolong the lives of women.

Traditional male gender roles and norms of masculinity encourage behaviours that pose serious risks to health and increase the likelihood of an early death (Sabo & Gordon 1995). Major accidents are far more common amongst men, as are fatal workplace injuries (principally because men predominate in high-risk industries such as construction, transport and manufacturing) (HSE 2002). Men are far more likely than women to experience risks to health and early death from the consumption of alcohol and illegal drugs. Thirty-eight percent of men, compared to 15% of women reported hazardous drinking in 2000; 13% of men and 8% of women reported using illicit drugs (ONS 2001b).

Many of these risks cluster among younger age groups. Men aged between 16–24, for example, have a substantially higher risk of work-related injury than older men (HSE 2002). Alcohol and drug misuse are among the major risks for suicide, now the commonest cause of death among young men in Britain (Chapter 9). There is a marked gender difference in suicide: between 1982 and 1996, male rates rose by 2.3%, compared to a decrease of 41.3% for females. Among 15–24 year old males there was a massive 102% increase in suicides over the same period (Men's Health Forum 2002). This has been linked to men's relative inability to express emotions and their tendency to externalise problems, often through physical aggression towards themselves and others.

Just as male gender roles lead to the risk of an early death, female gender roles are less likely to expose them to dangerous environments and less likely to lead girls and women to engage in risky behaviours that damage their health. Gender expectations mean that women are much less likely to drink alcohol at hazardous levels, to take illegal drugs, or to risk their lives through reckless driving and dangerous sports. While women are undoubtedly exposed to an array of health risks at work, these are less likely to be the kinds of hazards that lead to death from accident or catastrophic injury. Women's longevity may thus be related to their more positive health behaviour. Health-related behaviours are themselves part of building a particular gender-identity. For women, attention to health and the body helps to define femininity (e.g. through managing diet in relation to body size). There is evidence that women may be more likely to follow healthy diets than men, although they are also at greater risk of eating disorders such as anorexia nervosa and obesity. For men, excessive drinking and aggressive driving may be an integral part of their identity as 'real men'.

Use of health services

It is possible that women's greater use of health services may help to explain their longer life expectancy. It has been suggested that women make greater use of health services because they are more likely to recognise symptoms of illness and to seek medical help for health problems at an earlier stage than are men. This may be because women are more attuned to bodily changes (for example, the menstrual cycle, pregnancy) and it is more acceptable for them to ask for help.

The difference in the use of services is most clear-cut with respect to medical general practice. In 2000, 16% of women and 12% of men reported consulting a general practitioner (GP) during the two weeks prior to interview. Women's higher use of GP services is related to reproductive health (visits for birth control or pregnancy) as indicated by the fact that the largest gender difference is found among the 16–44 age-group, where women were twice as likely (16%) as men (8%) to have seen their GP (ONS 2002). Taking visits for reproductive health out of the equation reduces but does not erase the gender difference in GP visits. Gender differences in the use of other health services, such as hospitals, are less clear-cut and harder to interpret.

While women's earlier and more frequent use of GP services may contribute positively to their health, there is also some evidence that gender bias in medical consultations may counteract this. For example, women are less likely to be routinely tested for cardiovascular symptoms and are more likely to suffer unrecognised heart attacks than men. Studies show that women who go to their doctor with severe symptoms are not as likely as men with lesser symptoms to be given a coronary arteriography, catherisation, or bypass surgery (Sharp 1998).

It has been argued that men are less likely than women to recognise or seek help for illness because independence and stoicism in the face of pain are defining features of masculinity. Illness and injury are often seen as a kind of weakness to be overcome rather than given in to, for example 'rising above pain' and continuing to play contact sports when injured (Sabo & Gordon 1995). This has led to the suggestion that if men were to heed health education messages, for example being 'sun safe' to protect themselves against skin cancer (an increasing cause of death among males), and made greater use of health services this would improve their life expectancy. Health education and health promotion activities by practice nurses and those in out-patient clinics may need to be sensitive to these gender variations.

Responses to the threats of reproductive cancers provide a good example of gendered differences to the use of health services. Women have been strongly encouraged to check themselves for the signs of breast cancer, the leading cause of cancer death for women, and to take up screening, with a 76% uptake in 2001 (ONS 2002). In contrast, far less attention has been given until recently to educating men to recognise the signs of prostate cancer, the third most common cause of cancer death for men, and testicular cancer, which has a rising incidence. There is an extensive lack of knowledge about these diseases among men. For example, in 1998 80% of men had never heard of the PSA blood test for prostate cancer (Luck *et al.* 2000).

In summary, gender expectations and behaviours seem to be important in explaining the different life spans of men and women. Masculinity encourages behaviour that makes men vulnerable to early death, while femininity may support behaviour that protects women from early death and promotes longevity. Masculinity and femininity seem to affect health-seeking behaviour in opposite ways although it is impossible to assess the specific contribution that gender differences in the use of health services makes to longevity.

The narrowing gender gap in mortality

The previous section has shown that gender differences in mortality are strongly related to gender roles and behaviours. For the whole of the twentieth century women outlived men (Table 5.1), an advantage that continues into the new century. However, the late 1970s/early 1980s saw the beginning of a new historical period characterised by the very slow reduction in the differential life expectancy between men and women. Table 5.1 shows that, even though both male and female life expectancy are still improving, men appear to have made swifter gains since the 1980s than women. This is expressed as 'years of life gained'. We can see that the average 'years of life gained' by men over the period 1980 to 1995 was 3.1 years, while for women it was 2.4 years. The projected figures for those born between 1999 and 2021 are 3.5 and 2.8 years for men and women respectively. If the difference in life expectancy between men and women continues to reduce by about one and a half years per generation, then in a hundred years' time men will be living as long as women. Breaking the data down by age shows that the 'extra years' come mainly from middle-aged and older men (roughly ages 55–70) living longer (Fitzpatrick & Chandola 2000).

Explanations based on gender roles suggest that for males these gains might best be explained by changes in gender roles and behaviours that advantage men's health and disadvantage women's health. Such changes are thought to result from the convergence of gender behaviours in which 'men have become more like women', and 'women have become more like men'. Many men are cutting back on harmful health behaviours while women are taking them up, and many men are now taking actions to protect and improve their health (Vallin *et al.* 2001). Given the very complex relationship between health behaviours, health and mortality, it is impossible to make direct links between most of these broad changes and the declining gender gap in all-cause mortality. However, the link between lung cancer and smoking, and the attitudes towards and knowledge about sun damage and skin cancer, provide two examples that suggest links between changes in gender-related attitudes and behaviour and changes in gender patterns of mortality.

Lung cancer and smoking

Figure 5.1 shows the trends in smoking for men and women in England between 1978 and 1998. Two points are important. First, the decline in smoking has been more marked amongst men than amongst women. About 44% of men smoked in 1978; this had dropped to about 28% by 1998. For women, the drop is less evident: about 36% smoked in 1978, declining to around 26% by 1998. Second, by 1998 there was very little difference in the percentage of men and women who smoked. The prevalence of smoking is highest among younger people, and it is younger women in particular who are taking up smoking. In 1998, 33% of young women aged 16–19 smoked, compared to 31% of men. At ages 11–15, 10% of girls and 8% of boys reported that they smoked regularly (DoH 2000).

There is clear evidence that smoking is part and parcel of women's movement away from traditional gender roles and out of the home and into the world of paid work. Certainly, as the World Health Organisation (Samet & Yoon 2001) put it, 'girls

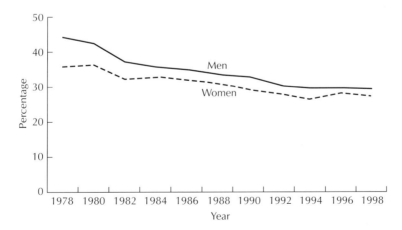

Fig. 5.1 The prevalence of smoking cigarettes among adults aged 16 and over by gender, England 1978–1998.
Source DoH (2000) Statistics on Smoking: England, 1978 onwards. *Statistical Bulletin* 2000/17. Crown copyright.

and women are being targeted all over the world by expensive and seductive advertising images of freedom, emancipation, slimness, glamour and wealth'. But although many women (and men) may be attracted to smoking in these terms, others turn to cigarettes as a way of coping with stressful lives. Graham (1994) found that 'smoking (was) one of the ways in which women handle and defuse the contradictory pressures that structure their lives', for example managing the combined pressures of caring for the family and holding down a demanding job. Working class women in particular 'survive by smoking' (Chapter 2). Women's increased smoking is therefore likely to be as much about the current socio-economic circumstances of their lives as it is about new-found 'freedoms'.

Cigarette smoking is estimated to be responsible for one in five deaths in Britain (DoH 2000). Thus, shifts in gender patterns of smoking are likely to be a major reason for the narrowing mortality gap. This can be appreciated by looking at changing patterns of deaths from lung cancer. Figure 5.2 shows that male deaths have always been and remain higher than female deaths. The timing of peaks and troughs in the incidence of lung cancer (the number of new cases within a time period) and mortality over time is quite different for men and women. For men, both incidence and mortality increased enormously from the early 1900s to reach a plateau in the early 1970s. Since then rates have declined. In contrast, for women both incidence and mortality increased up to the end of the 1980s. Since then both have remained fairly stable, rather than having fallen (ONS 2002).

These trends are a clear example of a cohort effect. Age cohorts refer to individuals born at the same time who are subject to similar environmental and lifestyle influences. The incidence of lung cancer increases with increasing age, reflecting the time lag between taking up smoking and the onset of the disease. Men at the

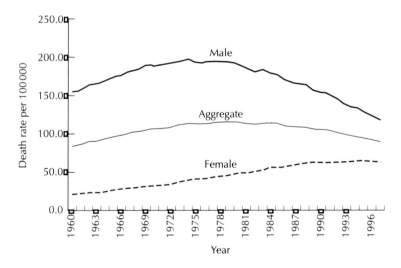

Fig. 5.2   Age-standardised lung cancer mortality rates by gender, England and Wales, 1990–1998.
Source   Willets, R. (1999) *Mortality in the Next Millennium.* Staple Inn, Actuarial Society, London. Reproduced with permission of the Actuarial Society, London.

highest risk of lung cancer were born in the 1890s, while women at highest risk were born in the 1920s, which was precisely the time when gender proscriptions on women's smoking began to lessen. This cohort effect in lung cancer deaths is likely to be a major contributor to the narrowing of the gender gap in all-cause mortality which, as Table 5.1 shows, began in the late 1970s/early 1980s. By this time women born in the 1920s would be around 60 years old and already subject to the negative health effects of smoking. Male smoking rates and lung cancer deaths were already declining by this time, especially amongst men in middle to older ages (ages 55–70), the male age cohort that has 'gained' most years of life in recent years.

Skin cancer

The evidence about gender patterns in lung cancer suggests a reversal of traditional gender roles that disadvantage women's health and life expectancy. Skin cancer presents the opposite picture, where changes in gender-related attitudes and behaviours are disadvantaging men. In the majority of cases skin cancer is caused by exposure to the sun's ultraviolet radiation. Its incidence has risen steadily for both men and women since the middle of the twentieth century, and has always been higher amongst women than men. However, despite its lower incidence, mortality has always been higher among men (i.e. men are less likely to get sick from skin cancer, but are more likely to die from it). Since the 1990s, skin cancer deaths have continued to increase for men, but have levelled off for women and at the start of the twenty-first century the gap between men's and women's incidence of skin cancer is the narrowest for 25 years. This is almost entirely due to increases among men. From 1982 to 1998 in England and Wales male rates increased by 12% and female rates by just 2.1% (Cancer Research UK 2002). Changing male attitudes may have influenced this rapid rise in skin cancer amongst men. In particular, body image is now much more important to men, especially young men, than it was in the past and 'getting a tan' is part of this. However, men are much less likely than women to see sun exposure as a serious risk to their health and less likely to heed 'sun-safe' messages. Although men and women are more or less equally aware of the health risks of sun exposure, women are far more likely to take action to protect themselves by the use of sunscreens and protective clothing, and far less likely to get sunburnt then men (ONS 1997). The changing patterns of mortality for lung cancer and skin cancer illustrate the ways in which the changing behaviour of women and men may play a part in converging mortality rates.

Morbidity: are women really sicker?

Although women live longer than men in Britain and other advanced modern societies, research has shown that they are sicker throughout their lives. While men tend to suffer from serious illnesses that cause early death, women live on with chronic, but not necessarily life-threatening illness. Thus women's 'extra five years' are typically not spent in good health. In terms of healthy life expectancy, that is years spent free of disability or chronic illness, women's advantage reduces to just two or three years (Acheson Report 1998).

Table 5.2 presents data on four measures of self-reported illness taken from the General Household Survey. It shows that for all ages combined, females report only slightly higher rates than males, with the exception of longstanding illness. However, a consideration of specific age groups shows varying gender patterns. For example, males in most age groups report higher levels of 'poor general health,' while females in most age groups report higher levels of 'restricted activity'. Longstanding illness is notable since it shows higher levels of chronic long-term illness in males than females in all but the oldest age group. For most conditions leading to a longstanding (chronic) illness there is no statistically significant difference between men and women. The main exception is musculoskeletal conditions (reported by 135 men and 161 women per 1000). The proportion of older women suffering from arthritis and rheumatism mainly explains this. At younger ages (16–44) men report higher levels of musculoskeletal conditions than women, perhaps reflecting the chronic health effects of sport-related injuries and accidents. Age-related gender differences also emerge for chronic respiratory problems, although here it is men who report higher levels at older ages (in these data, after age 44). For example, among those aged 75 and over, men were twice as likely as women to report respiratory problems (116 per 1000, compared with 58 per 1000) (ONS 2001c).

Table 5.2 Self-reported sickness: by type of complaint, gender and age (%) 2000–01, Great Britain. Crown copyright.

	Poor general health	Longstanding illness	Limiting longstanding illness	Restricted activity*
Males				
0–4	4	14	4	11
5–15	3	23	9	10
16–44	6	23	11	10
45–64	18	45	27	17
65–74	22	61	38	20
75 and over	29	63	44	23
All	11	33	18	13
Females				
0–4	3	13	4	7
5–15	3	18	8	11
16–44	8	22	11	12
45–64	16	42	27	19
65–74	21	54	35	21
75 and over	26	64	48	27
All	12	32	19	15

*This refers to whether respondents had cut down on their normal activities in the two weeks prior to interview.
Source Social Trends 35, Table 7.2.

The overall picture the data presents is of similar broad self-assessments of health for men and women, but also of age differences for specific categories, some favouring men, others favouring women. This national picture is supported by research on local populations. Data from the West of Scotland (Macintyre *et al.* 1996) found that although the proportions reporting their health as 'fair' or 'poor' were higher among women, this was only statistically significant for those aged 18. For symptoms of 'minor' ill-health such as colds, flu, stiff and painful joints, and trouble with eyes, women's rates were only higher at age 39. However, symptoms of mental distress ('malaise'), such as problems with nerves, worrying, and always feeling tired were far more common at all ages amongst women than amongst men.

The finding that women tend to report higher levels of mental distress is mirrored in wider research. In 1993 and 2000 the Office of National Statistics carried out national surveys of psychiatric morbidity of people living in private households (ONS 2001b). In 2000, 19% of women and 14% of men between the ages of 16 and 74 were assessed as having a neurotic disorder. Neurotic disorders, or depression and anxiety disorders, are defined by a variety of symptoms such as fatigue and sleep problems, forgetfulness and concentration difficulties, irritability, worry, panic, hopelessness, and obsessions and compulsions, which are present to such a degree that they cause problems with daily activities and distress. The gender difference is largely due to higher rates of 'mixed anxiety and depressive disorder' among women (11%, compared to 7% among men), since the percentages suffering from other disorders were very similar. Women appear to experience more severe symptoms (18%) than men (12%). Men and women may express psychological problems in different ways. While women under stress tend to become anxious and depressed, men under stress are more likely to drink heavily, take drugs or become physically and sexually abusive (Busfield 2000). These kinds of behaviours have often been left out of health statistics, contributing to the impression that they are a form of deviance, rather than an expression of mental ill-health. It should be noted that these stereotypically gendered forms of expression may be diminishing in con-temporary Britain. Heavy drinking is increasing among women and there is some limited evidence of increases in male rates of depression, which may be linked with the rise in male suicides (Shajahan & Cavanagh 1998).

The evidence presented above suggests that gender differences in overall levels of morbidity are mainly attributable to higher levels of female morbidity for minor symptoms and some kinds of mental disorders. The gender differences in long-standing illness do not represent higher overall levels of sickness among women, but vary by condition. Thus it is important not to assume that women experience higher morbidity levels for all conditions. Although it seems to be taken for granted in much research, the excess morbidity of females is far from an unproblematic and universal finding (Lahelma *et al.* 2001).

Early research on gender and health was very much concerned with women's health, for example the different experiences of health amongst 'housewives' and women who worked outside of the home. It was not until the late 1980s that there was much research directly comparing men and women (Annandale & Hunt 2000). Indeed, the possibility that *men's* experience is also influenced by gender norms and that this may affect their health was almost totally ignored until this time, since 'gender' was treated as synonymous with *women's* health. Even when men's health was brought into the picture, there was a tendency, which continues today, for researchers to make assumptions about the aspects of men's and women's lives that are important for their health *prior* to conducting their research. For example, conditions of paid work have been assumed to be important for men, while juggling home and work, caring for the family and supporting others have been assumed to be important for women. In making these assumptions, research placed men and women into traditional gender roles and experiences, regardless of whether this was in fact the case. Moreover, it was assumed that it was the *differences* between men and women that were important rather than any *similarities*, so the latter were overlooked or disregarded. For example, Macintyre *et al.* (1996) report that when they presented a research paper highlighting the fact that higher female morbidity is not universal, several listeners told them afterwards that they too had not found the 'expected' gender differences in health in their research. They had never drawn attention to it because they assumed it was due to a peculiarity in their research sample, rather than a real finding.

Although there may be aspects of women's lives in general that predispose them to higher levels of illness, and aspects of men's lives that predispose them to lower levels of illness, it is important not to be not blinded to similarities across gender and to differences within men and within women, for example differences by age (Chapter 6) and social class (Chapter 3).

Explaining gender patterns

One difficulty in interpreting gender patterns in morbidity is to decide whether the similarities and differences that are reported are accurate reflections of men's and women's health status. One concern is that rather than reflecting real health differences in sickness between them they may simply be artefacts, that is a reflection of the ways that men and women think about and act upon their health.

Research on gender and health has traditionally emphasised women's higher morbidity. Two competing explanations have been put forward. The first explanation is that their higher morbidity is real and a product of their poor socio-economic circumstances. This explanation draws upon the well-documented finding that people in poorer socio-economic circumstances tend to have the worst health (Chapter 3). It argues that since in general women tend to be in worse socio-economic circumstances, with lower incomes, fewer assets and resources, their health will suffer. This analysis also suggests that men's better health is real and a product of their better socio-economic circumstances. The opposing explanation is that the health statistics simply reflect the propensity for women to *over-report* ill health and for men to *under-report* ill health. This could occur in self-reports, the main source of national data in Britain, and also in the assessments that others, such as health practitioners, make about the health of men and women.

This second explanation draws on the presumed effects of gendered expectations of masculinity and femininity. If male stoicism and machismo lead men to deny illness, then they are less likely to report illness in interviews and less likely to go to the doctor and to appear in health service statistics. Conversely, the feminine 'caring role' is assumed to make women more attentive to bodily discomforts, more willing to seek help and more willing to adopt the 'sick role' (Verbrugge 1985), resulting in the inflation of women's ill-health statistics. The implication is that self-reported measures such as 'restricted activity' due to illness (as in Table 5.2) may be as much about gender-related behaviours in response to illness, as about levels of severity.

It is unsafe to take the amount of contact with health services as an accurate measure of the differences and similarities in men's and women's health. Health care providers, drawing upon gender stereotypes, may have different expectations about the health of men and women. Thus, they may be more likely to diagnose some conditions in men and others in women. This is especially likely when the presenting symptoms are vague and a range of possible diagnoses is possible. Indeed, it is precisely the milder forms of 'nebulous' illness, such as minor physical symptoms and neuroses, which permit greater discretion in terms of the perception, reporting of symptoms and their diagnoses that show a female excess. This adds weight to the argument that the reported female excess morbidity is an artefact for at least some conditions, especially mild mental disorders.

Much of the debate about whether gender patterns of morbidity are real or artefactual has been driven by concern about the possible inflation of women's ill-health. If women are being inappropriately labelled as sick, then this creates the impression that they are vulnerable, weak and incapable. This in turn could lead to their exclusion from social positions, such as well-paid but demanding jobs, which benefit health through improved self-esteem and high financial rewards. The reverse is also true: if men's ill-health is under-reported and generally neglected, then their health problems are likely to be denied, leading to unnecessary suffering as they 'soldier on' regardless (Men's Health Forum 2002). These negative consequences of gendered responses to illness for men have often been neglected because attention has typically been directed at the apparently higher levels of morbidity amongst women.

Gender, health and social change

Gender differences in mortality and morbidity in contemporary Britain reflect the interaction of biological differences between women and men and patterns of social change. For example, the narrowing gender gap in mortality is related to changes in circumstances (such as kinds of employment) and behaviour (such as smoking) that began several decades ago and are now affecting men and women in middle and older age. More recent changes in lifestyles and health-related behaviours of males and females, especially among younger age groups, are influencing contemporary patterns of sickness. These changes result from fundamental changes within British society (Chapter 10), especially in the socio-economic, educational, employment, domestic and leisure circumstances of women and men.

In Britain men have traditionally had greater access to education and paid employment than women and consequently have had greater economic independence. This was particularly marked during the 1950s and 1960s when it was usual for men to go out to work and for women to stay at home and care for children. It was during this period that sociologists first began to refer to 'gender roles', seen as social 'scripts' for how a man and a woman should behave and the attitudes that they should hold (Annandale 1998; Charles 2002). However, in contemporary Britain expectations of what it means to be a man or a woman are no longer as clear-cut as they once were. Probably the most important single factor leading to these changing gender roles and behaviours is changes in employment. In Britain traditional areas of male employment such as heavy industry and manufacturing have been in decline since the second half of the twentieth century. This has been accompanied by a rise in the female-dominated service sector (e.g. retail, banking, financial services and the leisure industry). As women's economic activity rates have risen, male activity rates have declined and there is now an almost equal gender balance in the workforce (Chapter 10). This change has had *direct effects* upon mortality through reductions in male deaths from work-related accidents. However, at least as important are the *indirect effects* upon health and morbidity through gender-related changes in lifestyle such as those indicated above.

There used to be a very strong association between the kind of work that people did and the lifestyles that they led. The new service economy is changing this by actively breaking down barriers between the consumption and lifestyles of what were once clearly defined and tightly bound social groups. Consumerism allows the expression of lifestyles and identities which are no longer tied directly to class and gender (Charles 2002). The boundary between work and home, once firmly entrenched for men as they kept their work and home life separate, is blurring, as home and the family become the centre of consumption. Conversely, women, once largely confined to the 'housewife' role are experiencing the separation of home and work through their paid employment in a working life outside the family. This is not to say that men and women are necessarily becoming *equal*. For example, there is still a substantial gap in income. Nor is it the case that men's and women's attitudes and behaviours are becoming *the same*. Rather, gender expectations are now less fixed and both men and women can engage in behaviour previously confined to the other gender.

The rising incidence of skin cancer amongst men provides an example of the result of the interaction of 'new' and 'old' forms of masculinity. The 'new' expectations of the desirable/healthy looking tanned body, previously a female preoccupation, work alongside 'old' feelings of invulnerability which lead young men to ignore the need to protect themselves from sun. For young women the benefits to health from their 'new' social and economic independence, linked to better educational qualifications and entry into the labour force, may be cancelled out by opportunities to engage in dangerous behaviours usually associated with earlier death for men. The substantial major increase in young women's consumption of alcohol (Alcohol Concern 2000), a direct contributor to death from liver disease and accidental death, and a major contributor to heart disease, breast cancer and upper digestive cancers, is a good example of this. This has been strongly associated with the stresses and strains that women experience as they juggle 'traditional' female responsibilities for home and family and new expectations of success in a 'male world'.

Recognising that there are *similarities* between men and women as well as differences, leads us to appreciate that men and women are not homogenous groups. There are also *differences within* genders, with substantial differences in gender-related behaviour by age. The convergence of gender roles, experiences and behaviours is more likely among younger men and women. For this reason, it is more appropriate to refer to masculinities and femininities in the plural, than to masculinity and femininity in the singular. For example, sociologists have suggested that it is one form of masculinity, the 'traditional' ('macho') form of masculinity, often called hyper-masculinity, which is particularly negative for men's health (Sabo & Gordon 1995).

Gender differences in health have broad implications for nursing practice. Gender-related attitudes and experiences influence the ways in which men and women view their health, their health-related behaviours, and the ways in which they act upon health problems. It is important that nurses take this into account when assessing and treating patients; but it is equally important not to expect patients always to act in gender-stereotypical ways. Feminist sociologists have for a long time pointed out that this can lead to misdiagnosis and inappropriate treatment. Examples of this are misdiagnosing a woman's symptoms of physical ill-health as 'psychosomatic' because women's problems are seen to be 'all in the mind', or misinterpreting the symptoms of a heart attack because heart attacks are thought to be a 'male disease'. However, it is important not to exaggerate these differences, particularly amongst young people, as gender roles and attitudes are becoming more fluid. It is important to appreciate that there may be as many similarities in health and health behaviour between men and women as there are differences. Equally, there are differences within men and within women. For these reasons while nurses need to be alert to the potential relevance of gender influence upon illness and health behaviour, they must also recognise that these may present in a variety of complex ways and are likely to be influenced by age, socio-economic status and ethnicity.

Summary

This chapter has argued that gendered patterns of mortality and ill-health in contemporary Britain are more complex and less clear-cut than was previously assumed. For mortality, the gap in life expectancy between men and women persists but appears to be very slowly narrowing. For morbidity, considering general measures of morbidity for all ages together, gender differences are small or non-existent, but some differences are seen for specific conditions at particular ages. It is unclear whether the reported patterns of morbidity have always been more similar than they seemed since differences reported in the past may have been an artefact of the kinds of questions that were asked and/or the failure to report similarities. If men's and women's patterns of death and ill-health are, as it seems, becoming more similar in contemporary Britain this is likely to be the consequence of the different experiences of men and women born into different age cohorts. For young people in particular, gender identity is likely to be negotiated in ways that open men and women up to experiences that both protect and undermine their health in complex and perhaps competing ways. This does not mean that gender is less relevant for health and illness, but that it may not longer operate in the clear-cut way that it once did.

References

Acheson Report (1998) *Independent Inquiry into Inequalities in Health*. The Stationery Office, London.

Alcohol Concern (2000) *Women and Alcohol – A Cause for Concern*. www.alcoholconcern.org.uk

Annandale, E. (1998) *The Sociology of Health and Medicine*. Polity Press, Cambridge.

Annandale, E. & Hunt, K. (2000) Gender inequalities in health: research at the crossroads. In: *Gender Inequalities in Health* (eds E. Annandale & K. Hunt). Open University Press, Buckingham.

Busfield, J. (2000) *Health and Health Care in Modern Britain*. Oxford University Press, Oxford.

Cancer Research UK (2002) *Experts warn of skin cancer 'time bomb' as cases continue to rise*. http//www.cancerresearchuk.org/press/pressreleases/sunsmart. Accessed July 15th 2002.

Charles, N. (2002) *Gender in Modern Britain*. Oxford University Press, Oxford.

Courtenay, W. (2002) A global perspective on the field of men's health: An editorial. *International Journal of Men's Health*, **1**, 1–14.

DoH (2000) Statistics on Smoking: England, 1978 onwards. *Statistical Bulletin* 2000/17.

Fitzpatrick, R. & Chandola, R. (2000) Health. In: *Twentieth-Century British Social Trends* (eds A.H. Halsey & J. Webb). Macmillan, Basingstoke.

Graham, H. (1994) Surviving by smoking. In: *Women and Health* (eds S. Wilkinson & C. Kitzinger). Taylor and Francis, London.

HSE (2002) *Levels of Trends in Workplace Injury: reported injuries and the Labour Force Survey*. Stationery Office, London.

Kraemer, S. (2000) The fragile male. *British Medical Journal*, **321**, 1609–1612.

Lahelma, E., Arber, S., Martikainen, P., Rahkonen, O. and Silventoinen (2001) The myth of gender differences in health: social structural determinants across adult ages in Britain and Finland. *Current Sociology*, **49**, 31–54.

Luck, M., Bamford, M., & Williamson, P. (2000) *Men's Health. Perspectives, Diversity and Paradox*. Blackwell Science, Oxford.

Macintrye, S., Hunt, K. & Sweeting, H. (1996) Gender differences in health: are things as simple as they seem? *Social Science and Medicine*, **42**, 617–24.

Men's Health Forum (2002) *Soldier it! Young Men and Suicide*. Men's Health Forum, London.

ONS (1997) *Health in England 1996*. Stationery Office, London.

ONS (2001a) *Cancer Trends in England and Wales 1950–1999*. Stationery Office, London.

ONS (2001b) *Psychiatric Morbidity among Adults, 2000*. Stationery Office, London.

ONS (2001c) *Living in Britain. Results from the 2000/01 General Household Survey*. Stationery Office, London.

ONS (2002) *Social Trends 35*. Stationery Office, London.

Pollard, T. (1999) Sex, gender and cardio-vascular disease. In: *Sex, Gender and Health* (eds T. Pollard & S. Brin Hyatt). Cambridge University Press, Cambridge.

Sabo, D. & Gordon, D. (eds) (1995) *Men's Health and Illness: Gender, Power and the Body.* Sage, London.

Samet, J. & Yoon, S. (eds) (2001) *Women and the Tobacco Epidemic.* World Health Organisation.

Shajahan, P.M. & Cavanagh, T.J (1998) Admission for depression among men in Scotland, 1980–95: a retrospective study. *British Medical Journal,* **316**, 1496–7.

Sharp, I. (1998) Gender issues in the prevention and treatment of coronary heart disease. In: *Women and Health Services* (ed L. Doyal). Open University Press, Buckingham.

Shorter, E. (1982) *A History of Women's Bodies.* Allen Lane, London.

Vallin, J., Mesle, F. & Valkonen, T. (2001) *Trends in Mortality and Differential Mortality.* Council of Europe Publishing, Strasbourg.

Verbrugge, L. (1985) Gender and health: an update on hypotheses and evidence. *Journal of Health and Social Behavior,* **26**, 156–182.

Women and Equality Unit (2002) *Individual Incomes of Men and Women 1996/97 to 2000/01: a summary.* Stationery Office, London.

Further reading

Annandale, E. & Hunt, K. (eds) (2000) *Gender Inequalities in Health.* Open University Press, Buckingham.

Charles, N. (2002) *Gender in Modern Britain.* Oxford University Press, Oxford.

Hayes, B. & Prior, P. (2003) *Gender and Health Care in the UK. Exploring the Stereotypes.* Palgrave Macmillan, Bastingstoke.

Chapter 6
Health and Illness in Old Age

The relationship between health and ageing, and in particular the health of older people, is an important issue not only in the world of health services but also in the wider public arena. Appreciating this relationship requires an understanding of the links between biological and social aspects of ageing. Negative depictions of old age as a time of increasing illness and dependency often distort the ways in which ageing and old people are discussed in the mass media and in health and social policy debates. This chapter examines the nature of concerns about health, illness and old age and the implications of Britain's 'ageing society' for both older people and health services. It will:

- Define and discuss the concept of an 'ageing society'
- Describe the social position of old people in contemporary Britain
- Discuss patterns of health and illness among older people
- Discuss the biological and social aspects of ageing
- Discuss the health service care for older people

An ageing society

An ageing society is one in which the *proportion*, rather than the sheer number, of older people in the population is increasing relative to the proportions of young and middle-aged people. Between 1901 and 1991 there was a fourfold increase in the numbers of people over retirement age in Britain (Sutherland 1999). Although the numbers of older people in Britain will continue to rise it is important to take a balanced view of this change. The proportion of people over retirement age will increase during the first two decades of the twenty-first century from 21% to about 25% of the total population, a less rapid rate of increase than in the previous three decades.

The ageing of British society and the prospect of rising numbers of older people are often portrayed in newspaper reports and television documentaries as threats to the viability of the pensions and welfare system and therefore as an intolerable future burden on society (Mullan 2000). Public perceptions have tended to concentrate on the supposed problems caused by 'too many' older people. Instead of celebrating the rise in the numbers of long-living people as one of the great successes of health care and a consequence of rising standards of living, there have been gloomy predictions of the effects of the so-called 'demographic time bomb' on an already over-stretched care system. In health care concerns have focused on whether the health services of the future will be able to cope with ever-growing numbers of frail and chronically ill people.

The ageing of society is often seen as a direct result of older people living longer than they used to do. However, increased longevity among people who have already reached the age of 60 is only one factor in causing the development of an ageing society. Declining birth rates and changes in the ratio of young to old people are of equal if not greater significance. In twentieth century Britain the birth rate gradually declined (despite the mid- to late 1940s 'baby boom') and the lower percentage of children and young people in the population at the end of the century meant that the proportion of older people in the population increased. The trend towards living longer played a significant, but less important, part in creating the ageing society. Men who had reached the age of 60 towards the end of the twentieth century could expect, on average, to live for another 15.6 years, only two more years than men aged 60 at the beginning of the century. The rise in women's later life expectancy during the twentieth century was more marked. Women aged 60 at the end of the century could, on average, expect to live for more than another 20 years, compared to only 13 more years for women aged 60 in 1901, a gain of seven years (Victor 1994).

There have been marked fluctuations in the percentage increases of numbers of older people over the past 40 years. Table 6.1 shows that some of the sharpest increases took place in the 1970s and 1980s, especially at the older ages, rather than the recent past. The table also shows how historical rises and falls in birth and death rates work their way through to affect numbers of older people in the present. For example, in the 1990s there was a slight percentage *fall* in numbers of people aged over retirement age but under 74 years, and only a modest increase in the 75–84 age group, reflecting the historical impact of the Second World War and of low birth rates in the 1930s.

At the turn of the century, while just over a fifth of the UK population is over the state pension age (60 for women, 65 for men), a much more rapid rise in the numbers of very old people (aged 85 and over) is expected. This will become evident especially between 2030 and 2050 when the mid-twentieth century 'baby boom' cohort reaches very old age and the 'oldest old' (i.e. those over 85) are expected to

Table 6.1 Percentage changes in the elderly population by decade and age group (UK).

Age	1961–71	1971–81	1981–91	1991–2001	2001–11
60/64–74*	17	4	−2	−7	−9**
75–84	13	24	17	7	−2
over 85	40	25	46	24	14

*Women 60–74, men 64–74
**Age group 65–74 (women and men)
Source C. Victor (1987/1994) *Old Age in Modern Society*. Adapted from Table 6.3.

triple in numbers by 2050 (Sutherland 1999). The over-85s are already the fastest growing age group in other societies such as the United States. It is this projected rise in the numbers of over-85s that particularly worries health service planners. Although they will still form only a very small minority of the total population in the future, they are assumed to be a group that will continue to need a dis-proportionately high amount of expensive health care (Figure 10.3 page 184).

Older people in contemporary Britain

The 2001 Census found that for the first time people over the age of 60 (21%) exceeded children under the age of 16 (20%) as a proportion of the UK population. Just over 7% of the population were aged 75 or over and there was a big increase in the number of those aged 85 (1.1 million) who made up 1.9% of the population (as compared to 0.4% in 1951). In this age group women outnumbered men in the ratio five to two. For all minority ethnic groups the proportion of elderly people was 4%.

More detailed information about older people is provided in the results from the General Household Surveys (GHS) in 1998 (Bridgwood 2000) and 2000 (*Living in Britain* 2001). For the current generation of older people marital status has important consequences for their social support, sources of help and immediate care and social isolation. Although most older people maintain contact with friends and relatives on a regular basis those who are in good general health are more likely to make frequent visits to them and to maintain contact with neighbours. Visiting others and contact with neighbours decreases with age. Frequent visits from others to older people are associated with poor general health. People living alone are more likely to receive visits from others than those living with somebody else.

In 1998, men aged 65 or over (72%) were much more likely to be married than women (44%). Conversely, they were much less likely to be widowed, especially those aged 85 or over where 47% of men and 74% of women were widowed. Slightly over half of those aged 65 or over lived with their spouse and just over a third lived on their own. Living alone increases with age, especially among women. Eighty per cent of widowed people live on their own. For older people living in their own home, their spouse and families (especially daughters) are the main source of practical and emotional support. Older people who are house-bound, over 85 and/or living alone are most likely to be receiving statutory and voluntary services such as home care, meals, community nursing or occupational therapy services.

About two thirds of older people owned their own home (compared to 68% of all households) and about a quarter lived in rented Council or Housing Association accommodation. One in ten older people living in the community were in sheltered housing, with a fifth of those aged 85 or over living in such accommodation. Over 90% of older people have central heating in their homes, a refrigerator and a tele-phone (98%). However, older people, especially those living on their own, are less likely than the rest of the population to own washing machines, microwaves, or tumble dryers and are much less likely to own video recorders or CD players or to have access to a computer in the home. Just over half of older people have access to a car or van, thus making them more likely to be dependent upon public transport.

About 4% of older people live in residential or nursing care homes, although the proportion of those living in these settings rises sharply with age. The *Health Survey for England 2000* reported that about a quarter of residents in care homes were aged 65–79, compared to about three quarters of those in private households. About a third of all people aged 90 or over live in care homes (Bridgwood 2000). Older women (76%) are much more likely to be living in care homes than older men (24%), but there is a more equal gender balance in households in the community (56% and 44% respectively).

Income levels among older people vary greatly, and reflect earlier socio-economic differences. Most people aged 65 or over will be primarily dependent upon a pension and those with occupational pensions are likely to be better-off than those depending upon a State pension. While the more affluent households are likely to be spending about a quarter of their income on food, heat, light and heating, the poorest households are likely to be spending about 70% of their income on these essentials (Vincent 1995). Of the approximately 10 million pensioners, 1.6 million receive income support, and even this under-estimates the rate of poverty among older people (Blakemore 2003).

It is important not to see 'the elderly' as a homogeneous group as there is great diversity among the elderly population of contemporary Britain. Patterns of household composition vary according to the age, sex and ethnicity of older people and the experiences of those who are old will be shaped by their socio-economic status and material resources, their religious and cultural values and beliefs, their ethnicity and their relationships with their families. Being old in contemporary Britain is a variable experience. As Tinker (1997) puts it, 'few people would attribute the same characteristics to a 30-year-old as they would to a 60-year-old. Why then should those in their sixties and in their nineties be classed together as one group?'.

Chronic illness, disability and healthy life expectancy

One of the most important sources of information about illness in older people is provided by the GHS. This asks a randomly selected sample of respondents about any illness or disability they may have and whether any longstanding illness limits the respondent's mobility, or restricts their ability to perform the necessary tasks of daily living, such as washing, bathing and domestic tasks. Table 5.2 (page 90) shows that ill-health increases with old age. In 2000–01 over 60% of people aged 75 or over reported a longstanding illness, nearly half reported a limiting longstanding illness and a quarter reported their activity was restricted.

As Table 6.2 shows, there is no conclusive evidence in the GHS that limiting long-term illness is becoming either markedly more or less common in older age groups. Comparing the years 1975 and 2000, for men in both age groups, and for older people as a whole, there was virtually no change in the incidence of limiting longstanding illness. However, for women a slightly lower rate was found in 2000. One difficulty in assessing such evidence is that it is mainly based on 'snapshot' comparisons of surveys of older people in different years. As yet there are no results from longitudinal surveys of health in older people in Britain that track the same cohort through time.

Table 6.2   Trends in chronic illness by sex and age, 1975–2000 (percentages in Great Britain reporting limiting longstanding illness). Crown copyright.

Sex/age group	1975	1991	2000
Men 65–74	36	40	38
Women 65–74	41	34	35
Men 75 and over	44	46	44
Women 75 and over	56	51	48

Source   Living in Britain: Results from the 2000 General Household Survey (2001) Office for National Statistics. Adapted from Table 7.1.

Limiting longstanding illness represents only one aspect of health and illness among older people. The *Health Survey for England 2000* reported that the prevalence of serious disability among those aged 65 or over was 16%, with a sharp increase with age for those living in private households. Serious disabilities were reported by 10% of those aged 65–79 and by 25% of those aged 85 or older. Over 70% of residents in care homes reported serious disability. The most common disability was locomotor disability, reported by about 30% of those in private households and 75% and 81% of men and women in care homes. This was markedly higher at age 80 and over, rising to 57% of women and 47% of men in private households. Disabilities negatively affecting personal care were much more common in care homes (58% and 66% for men and women) than in private households (14%). While sight and hearing deteriorate with age they are unlikely to involve severe disability for older people living in the community, although severe hearing disability in care homes was reported by 15% of men and 23% of women.

However, serious functional disability affects only a minority of older people at any given time (Bernard 2000). Whilst a considerable number are affected by limiting illnesses, about 80% of men and women over the age of 85 are able to feed themselves, bathe themselves, get in and out of bed, and use the toilet without help. Whilst these are relatively minimal requirements for the maintenance of independence and life satisfaction in old age, the great majority of the very old can still manage to meet them. Concentrating on the extent of illness and disability makes it easy to forget that at any point in time a large majority of older people are in relatively good health and are leading active lives.

Social class is very influential in determining patterns of health and illness (Chapter 3). The class inequalities in health that exist at younger ages persist and perhaps intensify in old age (Arber & Ginn 1998; Vincent 1995), as illustrated by the evidence in Table 6.3. This shows not only an appreciable divide in the amount of limiting illness between manual and non-manual groups, but also that the divide is wider among men in the over-65 age group (14% difference) than in the 45–64 group (10%). Caution is necessary in interpreting this information. Because it compares differences between two age groups (or cohorts) it cannot predict contrasts between future cohorts, which might show a reduction of class inequality. However,

Table 6.3 Percentages of older people aged 45–64 and 65 and over reporting limiting longstanding illness by sex and socio-economic status of household* in Great Britain, 2000. Crown copyright.

Non-manual/manual	Men		Women	
	Age 45–64	Age 65+	Age 45–64	Age 65+
Non-manual	22	33	22	38
Manual	32	47	31	44
All	27	41	27	42

*Socio-economic group of household reference person
Source   Living in Britain: Results from the 2000 General Household Survey (2001) Office for National Statistics. Adapted from Table 7.4.

it does suggest that class inequalities in health among men increase in later life. Conversely, it suggests an opposite trend among women, for whom there is less class inequality in the rate of illness in the over-65 group (6%) than in the 45–64 group (9%). The *Health Survey for England 2000* found that older people who had been manual workers were significantly less likely to say their health was 'good' or 'very good' than those who had been non-manual workers.

Table 6.4 provides an overview of the main types of illness experienced by older people in Britain. It shows that by far the major causes of chronic illness are the heart and circulatory system and the musculoskeletal system. The latter causes serious disabilities for about 10% of those living in private households and 65% of those in care homes (Health Survey for England 2000). Only a small pro-

Table 6.4 Chronic sickness: percentages* reporting longstanding illnesses, by age in Britain. Crown copyright.

Condition	65–74	75 and over
Heart & circulatory system	30	31
Musculoskeletal system**	27	31
Endocrine & metabolic	9	8
Respiratory system	7	8
Digestive system	6	6
Eye complaints	4	7
Ear complaints	3	5
Nervous system	3	3
Neoplasms	3	3
Mental disorders	2	2
Genito-urinary system	2	2
Average number of conditions reported by those with a longstanding illness	1.7	1.7

*Rates per 1000 were used in the source. Percentages have been rounded.
**Includes arthritis and rheumatism, back problems and other bone and joint problems.
Source   Office for National Statistics (2001). Adapted from Table 7.13.

portion of older people report longstanding illness resulting from neoplasms (cancers and benign growths). However, this underestimates the significance of cancers, as a cause of death in old age among both women and men. The death rate from cancer declines steeply from about 30% of deaths at age 65 to half that rate among men over 85, and to an even lower rate, slightly above 10%, among women (Sidell 1995). In addition to cancer, the other main causes of death in old age, heart disease, respiratory disease and stroke, are similar for men and women.

There are important differences between men and women in the sorts of illness that typically affect them, and these have implications for mobility, self-care and health service needs. Sidell (1995) observes that 'women pay a price for their increased longevity in terms of increased levels of non-life-threatening but highly symptomatic diseases such as arthritis'. She points out that, with some important exceptions such as diabetes, respiratory conditions and genito-urinary illnesses, the leading illnesses among older men tend to *decrease* with age. Conversely, women's health problems, e.g. heart disease, high blood pressure, stroke, and sight problems, tend to increase with age.

Healthy life expectancy

It is important to know how *healthy* older people are likely to be in the future. The concept of 'healthy life expectancy' suggests that we consider not just the extra years of life to be expected by the average person, but how many of those years will be free of a limiting long-term illness or serious disability. There is debate about whether the longer lives of older people are associated with an 'expansion' of morbidity (Gruenberg 1977) or its 'compression' into a relatively short period of time at the end of life (Fries 1980, 1989). Both patterns are evident in contemporary Britain. Some old people experience healthy life well into old age, whereas others spend their longer lives with longer periods of painful and distressing symptoms and disability. There are significant differences in patterns of health and disease in later life between men and women (Chapter 5) and between different ethnic groups (Blakemore & Boneham 1994).

The pessimistic view

There are several reasons to be cautious about taking an overly optimistic view of health and ageing. First, the evidence about the nature and extent of chronic illness and disability among older people reviewed above does not provide any conclusive evidence that illness is becoming markedly less common in older age groups, nor that it is being compressed into a short period at the end of life.

Second, the socio-economic inequalities in health discussed in Chapter 3 continue, and are exacerbated, in old age. A healthy old age and the compression of morbidity is most likely to be found among relatively affluent older people entering old age in good health; older people in poorer social groups are likely to experience increasing illness and disability throughout later life. Healthy old age for the latter therefore depends to some extent on the success of social and health policies in improving or maintaining health in the poorer sections of society, or in turning back the tide of rising social and economic inequality.

Third, there is no guarantee that succeeding generations of people who are now in their youth or young adulthood will continue the trend of continuous health improvement witnessed so far. Threats to children's and young people's health are causing concern, as evidenced by reports on obesity in young people, lack of exercise, smoking and drug use. It is possible that in the future the onset of heart disease, cancer and other serious illnesses will occur much earlier in the life course in significant numbers of people, rather than being compressed into a late life phase.

Another reason to be cautious lies in the subjective nature of illness. Despite growing social divisions, material living standards and health have improved steadily in Britain over the past few decades. But while health might continue to improve in the future, there is a strong possibility that people's *expectations* of health in later life will continue to rise faster than actual improvements (Chapter 10). The present generation of older people seem to be prepared to put up with a certain amount of illness and accept some chronic conditions as an inevitable part of growing old. However, future cohorts of older people may be much less likely to do so. It seems likely that the next generation of older people will report illness more frequently and expect more expensive and sophisticated treatments than those that are accepted today.

The optimistic view

The classic study by Fries (1980) suggested that the more that people enter later life in a relatively healthy state, the more likely it is that they will continue to enjoy a significant number of years in old age without chronic illness or disability. The population cohort now in their sixties will be the first in the UK to have grown up receiving universal health care, wider education opportunities, better nutrition and an improved standard of living compared to the cohorts that grew up before the advent of the welfare state in the 1940s. Thus, according to Fries, they should benefit from a healthier old age than their predecessors. It remains to be seen how much difference the impact on later life of improved socio-economic conditions and better health at younger ages will make, although it should not be assumed that the effects will inevitably be positive.

According to Sutherland (1999) the 'best evidence' is that the social and environmental improvements that have led to longer life expectancy are also leading to an increase in years of life that are free of serious disability. In the UK Victor (1991) compared data on health and illness in different age groups over time and found a lower amount of chronic illness among older people in the more recent cohorts. Manton *et al.* (1995) provide evidence from the US that disabling conditions among older people declined since 1982, especially for circulatory conditions. They estimated that the proportion of people aged 85 or over who remained free from disability increased by 30% between 1982–1989. In an Austrian study Doblhammer and Kytir (2001) found that both life expectancy and healthy life expectancy increased significantly over their 20-year study period.

Gruenberg (1977) and others have argued that improvement in medical treatments and preventive interventions have been an indirect contributor to rises in the total amount of illness, as better treatment allows more elderly people to survive and experience further illnesses. However, more recent evidence supports the view of Fries (1980, 1989) that these have helped to 'compress morbidity' into a relatively short period before death. Developments in pharmacological and surgical treatment, such as techniques to reverse neurological impairment and to prevent strokes, are already beginning to have a positive impact on the effects of long-term illness in older people (Dalley 1998). Relatively inexpensive and routine surgical treatments that greatly improve mobility and sight appear to have particularly beneficial effects and reduce the dependency of older patients on further treatment or care services. Many elderly patients gain as much from, and recover as well as, younger patients from surgery and medical treatment (Mullan 2000). For example there is no age difference, in terms of post-operative illness or mortality, in outcomes following coronary bypass surgery or kidney transplantation. In sum, far from adding to future costs, early and effective medical care in old age tends to reduce health problems and to compress illness into a relatively brief terminal period.

The common perception of later life as a period of inexorable decline in health is thus open to question. Comparisons of illness rates between groups of very old people (over 85 years) and people in their sixties and early seventies show that rates are lower in the older group for some significant diseases (Mullan 2000). For example, various forms of cancer and heart disease peak in the 60–70 age group and become less common in later life. Those who live into their eighties and nineties are the people who have been selected out as survivors, and a significant proportion are in relatively good health until a year or so before death. It is expected that improvements in health among the 'young old' (as reported by Victor 1991) are likely to reduce the total burden of illness in the elderly population as a whole, and will compensate for rising need among the growing group of people aged over 85.

In their 'Debate of the Age', Age Concern (1999) strongly supported the optimistic view that the compression of morbidity was reasonable, and that this could be achieved in contemporary Britain. They recommended that 'the compression of morbidity should be adopted as an explicit objective of health policy' and suggested that preventive and rehabilitation strategies should work alongside clinical research and improved practice to achieve this.

Ageing and health in older people

Discussion about rates of illness and death in the older population focuses on a rather medicalised view of later life. However, ageing is not merely a process of biological change, it is also a process of social change. To understand the role of nursing and of health services in the lives of older people we must take into account both of these aspects of ageing.

The bio-medical model of ageing and health

The bio-medical model of ageing is widely used and understood by nurses and other health professionals, and the general public. It focuses upon the ageing individual, and views human ageing as a process of physiological and biological change. Ageing is seen as being determined by an in-built biological process (a 'biological clock') programmed by our genetic make-up that governs significant bodily changes from early development to maturity through to the decline and loss of functions in later life. Ageing means an inevitable loss of health, and represents a decline from optimum levels in youth. Life stages – infancy, childhood, puberty and adolescence, adulthood and maturity, and old age – are predetermined. Although individuals may vary in the chronological age at which they enter and leave each stage, normal development includes passage through all the stages. Human behaviour and physical and mental health are strongly influenced by these stages and as individuals age they take on the characteristics of their biological age group, leaving behind the behaviour and interests of the earlier stages.

The bio-medical model focuses on the 'mechanical' processes of ageing. Different parts of the body such as knee and hip joints, the heart and liver, may age at different rates, much as different components in a car might fail sooner, or last longer, than expected. Thus, some of the negative aspects of physiological ageing are 'fixable', to a degree, by medical intervention. From this perspective old age comes to be seen as a form of disease or a complex of conditions that are treatable. But this optimistic view of the ability of medicine to intervene positively into ageing exists in tension with the underlying, more pessimistic, view that physical decline in later life is inevitable.

The social model of ageing and health

The social model of ageing emphasises the importance of social factors in shaping people's experiences of growing old. It suggests that both the ageing process itself and how it is viewed in a society are shaped by socio-economic conditions and cultural values throughout the life course (Chapter 3). While ageing is a biological reality, it is influenced by social and economic factors. Both health and the average life span have improved very significantly in industrial societies since pre-industrial times, and life expectancy is greater in today's industrial developed economies than in most poorer countries. In contemporary Britain and similar societies what is regarded as the 'natural', biological life span has been revised upwards.

As people age they tend to carry their health experience and their identities with them, rather than changing fundamentally at each stage, as the medical model suggests. As each cohort ages, it is likely to experience social, cultural and economic influences that are specific to their historical time. Thus, tomorrow's cohorts of older people are likely to be different in significant ways from those of today. For example, they might be more assertive and 'consumer minded' in their expectations of nursing and health care. Instead of seeing an older person's behaviour or health simply as a reflection of the physiological stage they have reached, it is important also to consider how the health of older individuals is influenced by the experiences of their age cohort (Chapter 3).

Health and illness in later life are influenced by the social roles older people adopt, as well by the physiological or 'mechanical' failure of different parts of their bodies. The social model draws attention to the important links between social role, bodily functioning and self-conceptions (Chapter 7). For many older people in contemporary Britain, especially men from lower socio-economic classes, entry to old age has been/is signalled by retirement from paid work and the receipt of a pension. Social arrangements and negative social attitudes in interaction with reduced income and increasing chronic illness may make it harder for some old people to participate fully in the whole range of 'normal' life. The social process of ageing may thus become marked by a progressive 'emptying out' of roles and activities and decreasing social integration within the wider community. This can have a detrimental effect on their morale, leading to lower performance of the immune system and physical illness. Conversely, valuing older people and recognising their worth can lead to better health, or at least to a more tolerable experience of illness. This has been found to be the case even with older people who have organic brain disorders such as Alzheimer's disease (Kitwood 1997).

The bio-medical and social models of ageing are best seen as complementing or informing each other, rather than as being in conflict. As the bio-medical model acknowledges, chronological age ('clock time') does not reliably predicate the onset and progression of disease in old age or the ability to benefit from treatment. Nor does it correlate reliably with the social activities, interests and aptitudes of older people. Taking account of the social aspects of ageing can lead to a better understanding of elderly people, their health and illness and their capacity to benefit from health care. For example, physical decline and social aspects of ageing such as the loss of meaningful or valued roles in work or family may reinforce each other, creating a negative effect on morale and physical health. The impact of illness is mediated by social support (Chapter 2). Older people with supportive social networks are likely to be less adversely affected by the same level of illness or disability than those who are socially isolated. Old age is thus best seen as a biologically based category that has been socially shaped and patterned. By understanding this, nurses may avoid the dangers of stereotyping old people and 'the elderly patient' as a single group.

Health care and older people

It is not clear how effective health services are in protecting older people against some of the hazards to health experienced in later life and in helping them to deal with their ill-health. While some older people benefit significantly from health care interventions for others deficiencies in their health care may compound their problems.

Preventive health care

The potential benefits of a preventive approach and of widening older people's access to inexpensive but effective forms of treatment have long been recognised in British government health policies. In 1978 the government issued a consultative document, *A Happier Old Age* (DHSS 1978) that stressed the benefits of both early detection of health problems in older people and rehabilitation to allow those who had been ill to avoid hospitalisation for as long as possible. The health reforms of the 1990s introduced a series of measures that were designed to improve preventive health care of older people such as requiring GP practices to monitor the health of all patients over the age of 75 annually. In 2000, both the NHS Plan (DoH 2000) and the National Service Framework for Older People (DoH 2001) made strong policy commitments to improving both preventive and rehabilitative services for older people.

Government achievements in preventive health care for older people have been very mixed in terms of their success. For example, the key policy document that was meant to renew the emphasis on prevention of illness and on the promotion of good health, *The Health of the Nation* (DoH 1991), was widely criticised for neglecting the health of older people (Dalley 1998). In terms of practice, there have been serious shortcomings in the extension of screening services to older people. For example, despite the policy initiative of *The Health of the Nation*, many health authorities in the 1990s did not automatically invite women aged 65 and over for breast cancer screening, even though incidence of that disease increases markedly among women over 60. Routine screening for cervical cancer was similarly denied despite 40% of deaths occurring in women aged 65 and over. While the benefits of preventive screening have perhaps been over-estimated, their relative lack of availability for the elderly illustrates the low priority given to the health care of older people.

The preventive strategies of both Conservative and Labour governments have emphasised the individual and behavioural determinants of health to the neglect of material and environmental influences, although the latter are now receiving more attention (Chapter 3). Hypothermia illustrates how a social or economic perspective is vital to a fuller understanding of what an effective preventive strategy requires. Hypothermia (having a core body temperature of less than $35\,^{\circ}$C) is much more common in older than younger people because in old age the human body has a decreased capacity to regulate temperature. Lack of heating in the bedroom, or low temperatures in the home generally, can easily lead to accidental hypothermia in older people. Despite the government's scheme of Winter Fuel payments to older people on low incomes the main cause of inadequate heating and insulation in the home is 'pensioner poverty'. In Sweden, which has much lower temperatures in winter than Britain, the occurrence of hypothermia is negligible because older people's standards of living and housing are high. Although there may be considerable benefits to a policy that helps to identify illnesses earlier and provides preventative and remedial treatment more effectively, raising the incomes of poorer old people above the minimum poverty level is likely to be more effective than any preventive health care strategy.

Use of services

The use of health services increases between the middle and later years of life and is particularly high among people aged 75 and over. There are a number of ways of interpreting older people's access to, and use of, the NHS. A major consequence of the development of community care in the 1990s was to reduce significantly the role of the NHS as a provider of long-term health care for older people and other groups (Ham 1999). The NHS now mainly concentrates on providing primary health services (through the GP service) and acute services. Many older people in need of long-term health and personal care can no longer use NHS hospital or nursing home services and instead must use a combination of services provided by local authorities and the private and voluntary sectors. This is of key importance in comparing the use of health services by younger and older age groups because a considerable proportion of the care (including nursing care) provided to older people now lies outside the NHS.

Whilst the differences between age groups in their *frequency* of use of health services are significant, they are not as wide as might be imagined. Table 6.5 shows that older men (75 and over) are seen by GPs at about the same rate as male babies and infants. However, older women see their GPs more often than young female

Table 6.5 Use of GP services and in-patient hospital services by selected age groups (1981/82* and 2000).

	Males		Females	
	1981/82	2000	1981/82	2000
GP consultations				
Average number per year				
Age 0–4	7	6	5	4
Age 5–15	2	3	3	3
Age 16–44	2	3	5	5
Age 45–64	4	5	4	5
Age 65–74	4	6	5	7
Age 75 and over	6	6	6	7
Percent consulting in the last 14 days				
Age 0–4	21	18	17	14
Age 5–15	7	8	9	9
Age 16–44	7	8	15	16
Age 45–64	12	15	13	16
Age 65–74	13	20	16	17
Age 75 and over	17	20	20	22
Hospital in-patient stays				
Percent in the last 12 months				
Age 0–4	14	8	12	6
Age 5–15	6	5	4	3
Age 16–44	5	4	15	11
Age 45–64	8	8	8	7
Age 65–74	12	8	13	13
Age 75 and over	14	18	12	18
All age groups	7	7	11	9

*GP consultations 1981; Hospital in-patient stays 1982
Source Office for National Statistics (2001). Adapted from Tables 7.18, 7.19 and 7.31.

children and are more likely to have seen a doctor in the previous 14 days. Overall, older people (aged 75 and over) use GP services more frequently than any other age group. This is particularly apparent when younger men (aged 16–44) are compared with men over 75, who are two and a half times more likely to have recently consulted a family doctor.

Looking at the use of in-patient hospital services, an equal percentage of older people and infants were hospitalised in 1982 but the percentage of young children admitted to hospital for in-patient services had dropped significantly by 2000. Despite the drive to reduce the numbers of older people in hospital, the percentage admitted fell only slightly among older men between 1982 and 2000, and remained the same among older women. This suggests that any reductions in use of in-patient services by older people have been achieved by reducing length of stay rather than the number of times older people are admitted to hospital. It is also likely that, as medical techniques have improved and some interventions have become more effective, both demand and need for hospital care have increased faster than population growth in the group aged 75 and over. Although there have been strong attempts by hospitals to reduce length of stay it is evident that not only is the frequency of hospitalisation greater among older people, but that length of stay remains appreciably greater. For example, the GHS shows that the average number of nights stayed in hospital as an in-patient rises with age, from five nights for 15–44 year olds to 16 nights for those aged 75 and over (ONS 2001).

In general, service use by older people, particularly those aged 75 and over, is appreciably greater than among young adults, although more so for in-hospital services than GP services. These patterns of health service use suggest that older people are not experiencing particular problems in terms of simple access to primary health care. For example, the GHS showed that almost a quarter of respondents aged 75 and over had received a home visit from their GP in the two weeks before the survey. This compared with less than a tenth of those aged 65–74 and only 1–2% of younger age groups (ONS 2001). Thus, despite difficulties in providing adequate GP services in some areas, most older patients are able to call a doctor to their home if they are physically unable to attend a surgery.

While access to primary health care services is not particularly problematic, research on older people's experience of the *quality* of both GP and hospital services has raised important questions. As Bernard (2000) puts it, 'high consultation rates do not necessarily ... translate into satisfaction with either services or professional responses.' Geriatric medicine is the specialty focussing solely upon older people. The development of a body of specialist knowledge and skills in the treatment of older patients has brought noticeable benefits to some, especially in the field of rehabilitation. It may also prevent inappropriately aggressive forms of drug therapy or surgery for older patients. However, there are also drawbacks to geriatric medicine. First, it has traditionally been seen as a low-status specialty by the medical profession and geriatric medical teams and departments have, as a result, often been less able than higher-status medical specialisms to attract enough staff and other resources to provide a satisfactory service. Secondly, it has sometimes played a significant role in diverting elderly patients from better and more prompt treatment in the health system by reinforcing the use of chronological age, rather than 'biological' age or medical need, to determine the services that are offered to older patients (Victor 1994). For example, older patients might be referred less quickly to specialists in the treatment of cancers and other life threatening diseases.

The effectiveness of the health care for older people seems to depend on the organisation of geriatric medicine and the degree to which it is integrated with other specialisms and, as Victor (1994) points out, there is considerable variation in this respect. In some health authorities, patients over a certain age are treated for a wide range of health problems by departments of geriatric medicine; in others, geriatric specialists are integrated with other specialisms. It is in the former type of arrangement that the potential for second-rate, segregated services for older people to develop seems greater, despite notable exceptions where first-rate treatments and after-care are provided to older patients through specialised centres (Swift 1989).

While accepting that older people are too often seen as the passive recipients of treatment and services, and that they are often disadvantaged in access to services, there is little evidence to suggest widespread overt discrimination against older people on the grounds of age (Dalley 1998). There may be agreement between doctor and patient to accept that symptoms that would lead to a fuller examination of a younger person are simply to be expected, and these are accepted by the older patient as part of the inevitable decline of old age. Further, many older patients may be anxious that younger adults, including nurses and doctors, will inappropriately take charge of their lives (Biggs 1993). Therefore it may seem 'safer' to some older patients to agree with the doctor who discounts a treatable illness as simply a problem of old age rather than precipitating a series of unwanted medical investigations and changes in the older person's life. However, older people often feel that doctors and other health practitioners have not listened to them and that they have not been given adequate explanations of their health problems or treatments (Bernard 2000; Sidell 1995).

Rationing health care for older people and limiting their access to services that are provided more readily to younger people can be seen as indirect forms of age discrimination. Concerns about the unspoken use of age criteria in a wide range of medical treatments, and in health services generally are regularly expressed in the British mass media. Direct age discrimination has been observed in the day-to-day work of nurses and doctors, and in the ways that health care is provided to older people (Bowling 1999). Although it is a major public concern, it is difficult to ascertain exactly how widespread ageism is in health (and social) care. However, the problem is perceived to be so significant that 'rooting out age discrimination' is one of the main targets in the National Service Framework for older people (DoH 2001).

Summary

In contemporary Britain the number and proportion of older people will continue to increase, a prospect that has alarmed health policy makers because of the anticipated consequences for the costs of health care. However, there is disagreement about whether the ever-extending lives of older people will result in longer periods spent in illness and dependency or whether they will be spent in healthy old age. Both the 'compression' of illness and longer years spent with illness and disability are evident in contemporary Britain. Becoming and being old is not a uniform experience but varies by generation, social class, ethnicity and gender. It is thus difficult to generalise about the relationships between health, illness and old age. It is, however, wrong to suggest that, at a given chronological age, every older person will be ill, frail and disabled, or have a well-defined range of health care needs. Nevertheless, older people will remain the largest users of health services for the foreseeable future. The effectiveness of these appears to be variable. The impact of health promotion and preventive strategies on health and life expectancy appears to be relatively weak, access to primary care and hospital services is generally adequate, although patchy, and indirect and direct discrimination on the grounds of age are evident.

References

Age Concern (1999) *The Future of Health and Care of Older People: The Best is Yet to Come.* Age Concern England, London.

Arber, S. & Ginn, J. (1998) Health and Illness in Later Life. In: *Sociological Perspectives on Health, Illness and Health Care* (eds D. Field & S. Taylor). Blackwell Science, Oxford.

Bernard, M. (2000) *Promoting Health in Old Age.* Open University Press, Buckingham.

Biggs, S. (1993) *Understanding Ageing: Images, Attitudes and Professional Practice.* Open University Press, Buckingham.

Blakemore, K. (2003) *Social Policy: An Introduction*, 2nd edn. Open University Press, Buckingham.

Blakemore, K. & Boneham, M. (1994) *Age, Race and Ethnicity.* Open University Press, Buckingham.

Bowling, A. (1999) Ageism in cardiology. *British Medical Journal*, **319**, 1353–5.

Bridgwood, A. (2000) *People aged 65 and over.* ONS, London.

Dalley, G. (1998) Health and social welfare policy. In: *The Social Policy of Old Age* (eds M. Bernard & J. Phillips). Centre for Policy on Ageing, London.

DHSS (Department of Health and Social Security) (1978) *A Happier Old Age.* HMSO, London.

Doblhammer, G. & Kytir, J. (2001) Compression or expansion of morbidity? Trends in healthy-life expectancy in the elderly Austrian population between 1978 and 1998. *Social Science and Medicine*, **52**, 385–91.

DoH (Department of Health) (1991) *The Health of the Nation: a consultative document for health in England.* HMSO, London.

DoH (2000) *The NHS Plan – A Plan for Investment, A Plan for Reform.* Stationery Office, London.

DoH (2001) *The National Service Framework for Older People.* Stationery Office, London.

Fries, J. (1980) The compression of morbidity: Near or far? *Milbank Memorial Foundation/ Health and Society*, **67**, 208–32.

Fries, J. (1989) Ageing, natural death and the compression of morbidity. *New England Journal of Medicine*, **303**, 130–35.

Gruenberg, E. (1977) The failures of success. *Milbank Memorial Fund Quarterly*, **5**, 1.

Ham, C. (1999) *Health Policy in Britain*, 4th edn. Palgrave, Basingstoke.

Health Survey for England (2000) *The Health of Older People*. National Statistics. The Stationery Office, London.

Kitwood, T. (1997) *Dementia Reconsidered*. Open University Press, Buckingham.

Living in Britain. Results from the 2000 General Household Survey (2001) The Stationery Office, London.

Manton, K.G., Stallard, E. & Corder, L. (1995) Changes in morbidity and chronic disability in the US elderly population: evidence from 1982, 1984 and 1989 National Long Term Care Survey. *Journal of Gerontology*, **50B**, S104–S204.

Mullan, P. (2000) *The Imaginary Time Bomb – Why an Ageing Population is not a Social Problem*. Tauris, London.

Office for National Statistics (ONS) (2001) *Living in Britain: Results from the 2000 General Household Survey*. The Stationery Office, London.

Sidell, M. (1995) *Health in Old Age*. Open University Press, Buckingham.

Sutherland, Sir Stewart (1999) *With Respect to Old Age: Long Term Care – Rights and Responsibilities*. Cm 4192-1. The Stationery Office, London.

Swift, C. (1989) Health Care of the Elderly: the Concept of Progress. In: *Human Ageing and Later Life* (ed. A. Warnes). Edward Arnold, London.

Tinker, A. (1997) *Older People in Modern Society*, 4th edn. Longman, London.

Victor, C. (1991) Continuity or change? – inequalities in health in later life. *Ageing and Society*, **11**, 23–39.

Victor, C. (1994) *Old Age in Modern Society*, 2nd edn. Chapman and Hall, London.

Vincent, J. (1995) *Inequality and Old Age*. UCL Press, London.

Further reading

Bernard, M. and Phillips, J. (eds) (1998) *The Social Policy of Old Age*. Centre for Policy on Ageing, London.

Mullan, P. (2000) *The Imaginary Time Bomb: Why An Ageing Society is not a Social Problem*. Tauris, London.

Part III
Illness and Dying

Chapter 7
Chronic Illness and Physical Disability

In contemporary Britain the main burden of disease comes from long-term chronic diseases. There are also many members of our society, especially among the elderly, who have longstanding physical disabilities. Most nursing work, both in hospitals and in the community, involves working with people who are chronically ill and who may have physical disabilities. Most chronic illness and physical disability is made sense of and treated within the bio-medical model of illness (Chapter 2). This offers explanations of underlying pathology and offers means of controlling or alleviating symptoms with varying degrees of success. Through the application of the bio-medical model our ability to manage chronic illness and physical disability has become more effective and the lives of sufferers extended and enhanced. However, to be ill is also to be in a socially altered condition and individual experiences of chronic illness and disability are shaped by wider social contexts. This chapter will:

- Outline definitions of chronic illness and disability
- Discuss the distribution of chronic illness and physical disability in contemporary Britain
- Examine the relationship between body, self and identity in chronic illness and physical disability
- Discuss factors influencing the experience of living with chronic illness and physical disability
- Discuss coping with chronic illness and physical disability and the role of others

Defining chronic illness and disability

Chronic illnesses are long-term conditions from which there is no possibility of a complete return to the pre-morbid state enjoyed by the individual before they became unwell. The physical changes in the body are permanent. The longevity of the experience of the person who is chronically ill means that they develop a degree of expertise in their own treatment (DoH 2001). It also means that because of their expertise, their involvement with their medical carers is different from those of people who experience acute episodes of illness. With many acute episodes of illness the sufferer may expect to recover fully following medical intervention. In contrast, most chronic conditions are continuous, but not stable and many worsen over time. Medical and nursing intervention, whilst alleviating symptoms, will not lead to full recovery. Sometimes chronic illnesses lead eventually to death or have life-threatening complications. However, it is important to remember that many chronic illnesses also have acute episodes. Some acute illnesses are not curable in the sense of a complete return to normal health being possible, and the typical human has episodes of biological disturbance on average about once a fortnight (i.e. chronically).

Physical disabilities are sometimes associated with chronic illness but may also result from acute illness, accidents or congenital conditions. The definition of disability is highly contested. The World Health Organisation (in 1980) attempted to distinguish between physical difference in the human body (say the loss of a limb), the particular problems that ensue in operating in the physical and social environment as a consequence of the physical difference, and the social responses of the world at large to these. In this classification impairment refers to any disturbance of the normal structure and functioning of the human body; disability refers to the loss of or reduction of functional capacity; and handicap refers to the social disadvantages that result from impairment or disability.

The bio-medical model (Chapter 2) tends to treat acute and chronic illnesses and physical disability in much the same way. The physical departure from a biological norm is the focus of therapeutic intervention, the purpose of which is either to return the acutely ill person to normal or to ameliorate in some way the physical problems of the person with a chronic illness or disability. Therapeutic actions based on a narrowly biological approach have been very effective in helping to manage chronic illnesses like diabetes, epilepsy, angina, and interventions like hip replacement surgery have helped many people regain a good quality of life. However, this approach has attracted criticism. Two different positions in opposition to the bio-medical focus may be identified: the sociological and the disability studies perspectives.

Over a forty-year period sociologists have developed a way of describing chronic illness that emphasises the importance of understanding the experience of living with chronic illness. They have noted that across a number of diseases similar sorts of experiences ensue which, in social and psychological terms are the same or very similar, independent of the underlying physical problem. A variety of behaviours have been identified. These include coping with changes in relationships with family, friends and workmates, reorganising life expectations, adjusting to the limitations imposed by the illness, and dealing with economic disadvantage and various degrees of discrimination. Sociologists emphasise that these experiences are social and cannot be understood or predicted on the basis of the bio-medical changes in the human body. Moreover, the problems attaching to the care of people with chronic disease are as much about the social and psychological consequences of the illness as about the physical needs emphasised in the bio-medical model (Strauss *et al.* 1984; Bury 2001)

Writers interested in disability have taken a more overtly political stance, arguing that to focus on the physical impairment not only misses the important dimension of the social experiences of the disability but, more importantly, hides the fact that it is society that *creates* disability. They argue that the institutions of society (e.g.

schools, work organisations, the legal system) are based on the wants and needs of able-bodied people and systematically discriminate against people who have disabilities. In addition, physical environments are designed for able-bodied adults, e.g. access to buildings are made more difficult by physical barriers. These social and physical barriers to integration, it is argued, are political matters amenable only to political solutions. The issue is one of power in society not of the physical impairment itself. Consequently, such writers view a bio-medical response which focuses only on therapeutic interventions and care, even when driven by compassion, as at best inadequate and at worst compounding the problem. They argue that the negative consequences of having a disability can only be overcome by transforming society itself (Oliver 1996; Priestly 1999).

Oliver (1996) summarises this socio-political model of disability as follows: '. . . it is society which disables physically impaired people. Disability is something imposed on top of our impairments by the way we are unnecessarily isolated and excluded from full participation in society.' While the WHO model sees a causal connection between chronic illness and the disadvantages disabled people suffer, the social model of disability asserts that the disadvantages of disability have little to do with the physical consequences of illness and impairment. A two-fold division betwen illness and impairment on one side and socially constructed and shaped disability on the other is posited. This division focuses attention upon disability as a long-term disadvantaged *social* state that is shaped by social and political factors. It is argued that the WHO scheme obscures this fundamental reality, by locating disability as a property of individuals, 'medicalising' it and implying that medical and other experts should 'treat' what is in fact a social product. This devalues and disempowers disabled people and may create and reinforce their unnecessary dependence upon others.

Chronic illness and physical disability in contemporary Britain

Estimates of the number of people with a disability in Great Britain vary according to the criteria used in defining disability and the research methods used (see Chapter 1). However, official statistics suggest that at the turn of the century some 17.5 million adults living in Britain suffer from a long-term condition and that 8.5 million people are disabled. Table 7.1 summarises some of the most common chronic and disabling conditions. Very significantly these are not spread randomly in the population but are patterned.

There are important inequalities in ill-health at all phases of the lifecycle (Chapter 3), and these continue into old age (Chapter 6). People from lower socio-economic strata as compared to those from middle and higher strata are more likely to experience chronic illness and disability, and are more likely to experience financial, domestic, and work-related difficulties as a result of their condition (Chapter 3). In addition to socio-economic status, the patterning of chronic illness and disability varies by age (Chapter 6), ethnicity (Chapter 4), gender (Chapter 5), geography, and environment. There are, in simple terms, much higher volumes of both chronic illness and disability, among the least advantaged. There are no significant

Table 7.1   Common chronic and disabling conditions in the UK.

Arthritis, in some form, affects about 8.5 million people, including about 14 500 children. Approximately half of sufferers are below and half above the age of 55. Above 75, women are nearly twice as likely as men to report arthritis and rheumatism.

Asthma is estimated to affect over 3.4 million people, including 1.5 million children aged 2–15. It is the most common childhood disease, and its prevalence is rising. It affects approximately a fifth of all teenagers.

Back pain is thought to be the most commonly reported type of pain. Back pain lasting more than a day in the previous 12 months was reported by 40% of adults in 1998. Fifteen percent of back pain sufferers said they were in pain throughout the year, and approximately 40% consulted a General Practitioner for help.

Blindness: there are nearly a million blind people in the UK, most of whom lost their sight gradually as they became older. In England 69% of those registered as blind or partially sighted in 2000 were aged 75 or over.

Bronchitis: chronic bronchitis increases significantly with age, especially for men. It is uncommon among those under the age of 40 but affects about 10% of those aged 60–85. Above 75, men are twice as likely as women to report chronic respiratory problems.

Cancer is commonly seen as a fatal disease. However, earlier detection and improved treatment mean that many cancers are becoming similar to other chronic conditions. It has been estimated that one in three Britons will eventually be diagnosed with cancer.

Coronary heart disease affects about 2.4 million men and 875 000 women, mainly those over the age of 55. Its prevalence increases sharply with age. Heart failure has been estimated to affect over half a million people.

Deafness: there are about 8.6 million deaf and hard-of-hearing people in the UK, about 673 000 of whom are severely or profoundly deaf. 20 000 children (0–15) are moderately or severely deaf, about half of whom were born deaf. Deafness and loss of hearing increase with age, with 55% of those over 60 being hard of hearing. A higher proportion of men than women are hard of hearing.

Diabetes Mellitus: there are at least 1.5 million cases of diabetes, but many cases remain undiagnosed. About 80% of diabetics are diagnosed in middle age or later with the non-insulin dependent form. Insulin dependent diabetes is most likely to appear in childhood, especially between 10–13 years.

Epilepsy is the commonest serious neurological disorder affecting more than 420 000 people or 1 in 130 of the population. Epilepsy can affect people at any age and from any walk of life.

Multiple Sclerosis is one of the most common diseases of the central nervous system. It is estimated to affect between 80–90 000 people. It usually strikes people when they are young adults. MS affects women more than men in the ratio 3:2.

Sickle cell diseases are inherited blood disorders that affect a significant minority of people in minority ethnic groups.

Strokes: over 80% of strokes occur in people aged 65 or older. About 88 000 people a year experience a first stroke and nearly 54 000 people experience a recurrent stroke. A quarter of men and a fifth of women can expect to experience a stroke if they live to the age of 85.

Compiled from a range of sources.

gender differences in the overall reported prevalence of common conditions, apart from musculoskeletal conditions where more rheumatoid arthritis among older women results in higher overall prevalence among women (250 women per 1000 compared with 131 men per 1000 aged 75 or over reported these conditions). However, gender related patterns are evident within diseases, especially in old age (Chapters 4 & 6).

Table 5.2 (on page 90) shows that there are significant variations in the pattern and distribution of chronic illness by age, with over 60% of men and women aged 75 or over reporting they had a longstanding illness. The number of people who experience longstanding problems and come to be defined as disabled in some way is increasing with the ageing of the population and the greater number of people living beyond 75 and 85 (Chapter 6). Between two thirds and three quarters of these will have one or more longstanding illnesses and consequent disabilities. This is three times the rate for those aged 16 to 24 (DoH 2001). Some of these conditions are treatable: cataracts, hip replacements and hypertension are good examples where long-term problems can be managed quite successfully, and where considerable disability can be alleviated (Bunker 2001). There is also a large volume of illness linked to heart disease and diseases of the circulatory system, respiratory diseases, and cancers, that are not so easily amenable to successful restorative intervention, and where the requirements for long term care accumulate in the population (Wanless 2001).

Athough many elderly people remain fit and active until very late in their lives, chronic illness and disability are common experiences for old people, especially among those over the age of 75. A typical progression would be to experience non-serious levels of reduced mobility, vision and hearing which do not threaten their autonomy and independence. These may gradually deteriorate into a situation marked by multiple pathology and disability which, although restricting, does not compromise independence. A further decline in health and increasing disability may lead an elderly person to become dependent upon others (usually their partner and family) for help with basic activities of living if they are to remain in their own home. Finally, this situation may break down, perhaps as a result of an episode of acute illness or an accident (such as a fall resulting in a fractured femur) that leads to hospitalisation and the long-term loss of independence. The effect of chronic illness and disability is mediated by the social support old people receive. Those who are isolated are likely to be more adversely affected by the same level of sickness or disability than those with supportive networks (Chapter 2), and are more likely to be admitted to nursing homes or hospitals.

The most recent detailed survey of disability among children in Great Britain (Bone & Meltzer 1989), found that there were around 360 000 disabled children. Among children with disabilities there were more boys than girls, a difference also reported in later General Household Surveys. The commonest types of disability were behavioural (affecting 2.5% of those aged 5–15), followed by disabilities in communication, locomotion and intellectual functioning. The rates in the area of behaviour declined after age 15, suggesting that 'it is likely that the very different questions asked about behaviour in children and adults are responsible for at least part of the difference'. Inherited blood disorders are chronic conditions that affect a significant minority of children and young people in ethnic minority communities (Chapter 4). Although levels of chronic illness among adolescents are lower than for adults, the proportion of self-reported longstanding illness or disability increased from about 12% in 1975 to 20% in 1998–99 among those aged 13–24 (Matheson & Summerfield 2000).

Chronic illness and physical disability have economic and social effects. People who are chronically sick or disabled may be unable to work, or can participate in the labour market in only very limited ways and in less well-paid work. Yet it is more costly to be chronically ill or have a disability than to be in normal health. Direct costs may be incurred through the alteration of the home to accommodate disability, more frequent laundry, special dietary requirements, additional heating costs, and the employment of additional help in the home. Indirect costs may also be significant as activity restriction may affect access to large (and cheaper) supermarkets and require the use of taxis. Not only may people with disabilities suffer loss of income through restriction or loss of paid employment, but their partner or other main 'lay carer' may have to give up their paid employment in order to look after the person. Loss of income and the increased costs of being ill or disabled are unlikely to be adequately compensated by the range of financial arrangements available through the welfare state systems.

These economic disadvantages are not simply an outcome of chronic illness or disability but may also reflect the social patterning of disadvantage (Chapter 3). That is, they are linked to preceding disadvantages that are a risk factor for the morbidity in the first place. For example, functional limitations and disability in young people are frequently the results of accidental injury. There is a five-fold difference in the rate of accidental injury between the top and lowest social classes in contemporary Britain (Millward *et al.* 2003). Accidents are not random events; they follow the contours of social disadvantage and are a striking example of the way that disadvantage is both cause and effect of chronic illness and physical disability.

Body, self and identity in chronic illness and physical disability

A useful way of thinking about the impact of an illness or a disability is to focus on their effects on the relationships or attachments which people have. Two aspects of the person that are central to understanding the experience of chronic illness and disability are self and identity. Our sense of self is our personal and private subjective sense of who and what we are, while our identity is the way other people publicly define and see us on the basis of our behaviour and appearance. Just as the body may be thought of as providing a physical 'thread' of continuity through life, despite its constant changes, the self provides a socially shaped sense of continuity through the life course. For most of the time there is a near congruence between the roles and statuses to which we aspire and play, and our own sense of who we are and the way that others respond to us. Our sense of self is normally relatively stable and enduring and only becomes an issue if our identity is mistaken, or some serious life event such as an illness causes us to question our place in the world and to rethink our sense of who and what we are. Changes in the appearance of the body and in its functioning resulting from chronic illness or disability may profoundly affect the way people think about themselves and their levels of self-esteem (Kelly & Field 1996).

One of the ways in which body, self and 'society' mesh in chronic illness and physical disability is through the technologies that are used to assist managing the restrictions on social life resulting from them. A range of technologies are now available that can facilitate:

- Communication with others
- Mobility
- Physical safety
- Control over one's body
- Independence
- Participation in work
- Participation in the community

In their qualitative study of people with disabilities Lupton and Seymour (2000) found that their respondents felt that their disabilities should not define their identities and that 'technologies were valued for allowing them to tame the disorderly aspects of their bodies and thus facilitate social integration'. Technologies that were 'normalising' integrated the user unobtrusively into social life and relationships (especially computer technologies) and were highly valued. Conspicuous technologies (e.g. wheelchairs) that highlighted the disability, although beneficial, also served to 'separate out' their users and were perceived more negatively.

Chronic illness and physical disability involve not simply the loss or change of functions or roles; they also have the potential to change the very sense that someone has of themself. Not only does their body function differently, but their normal roles and activities will also be disrupted. Their inability to walk or to exert themselves as much as previously may prevent them from continuing highly valued activities, leading to the diminution of social contacts and attachments at work, in their leisure activities and within their home life. In the face of persistent and continuously debilitating symptoms, they may have to come to terms with the fact that they will not work again, that they will not be able to play energetically with their grandchildren, and that they will not be able to make love to their partner with the passion and frequency that they did before they were ill, thus leading to a changed sense of self. Strong feelings and emotions may be aroused as people try to come to terms with the loss of their previous abilities and social roles and struggle to maintain positive feelings of self-worth. Indeed, Charmaz (1983) suggests that the 'loss of self' is a fundamental form of suffering for chronically ill people.

Medical diagnosis and entry to the sick role (Chapter 2) plays an important role in shaping the experience of chronic illness by creating an identity that guides the actions and interpretations of self and others. While sickness is unpleasant it is understood that in most circumstances the person who is ill retains at least some of the characteristics that they had before they were ill. In our earlier example, a person may not be energetic but still has important roles with their partner and grandchildren. Chronic illness and disability are different here in at least one very important respect. In the case of chronic illness the sick role often has a highly positive connotation, facilitating access to a range of potentially helpful resources. In particular, where the symptoms of the disease are ambiguous and take a long time to diagnose, e.g. multiple sclerosis, the eventual diagnosis may be received with relief because of the certainty and legitimacy it provides (Robinson 1988). However, many physical disabilities are not caused by illness and many disabled people are not ill, so their role is not easily defined within the frameworks provided by the sick role for the management of illness. While there may be some benefits for sufferers of the practice of treating disability as if it were a sickness, there are also disadvantages. Requiring the disabled person to assume the sick role in order to gain access to a range of benefits and services may both restrict their autonomy and lead to dependency.

Factors influencing the experience of chronic illness and physical disability

Onset of the condition

The way in which chronic illness and physical disability appears has a profound influence upon identity and coping. Three main patterns may be identified: the acquisition of disability(s) at birth or infancy, suddenly (perhaps as a result of an accident), or as a result of a lengthy period of chronic illness (Table 7.2).

Some people are born with their disease or disabling condition either as a result of a genetic condition (e.g. cystic fibrosis) or due to something going wrong during pregnancy or at birth (e.g. a neural tube defect leading to cystic fibrosis). Infants may acquire a disability through infections, for example deafness resulting from bacterial meningitis or measles. Research in the 1960s–1980s found that the initial problems associated with such disabling conditions mainly concerned the adjustment of the parents (e.g. Darling 1979), whose reactions have been described in terms of coping with loss. Nurses and other health workers may also experience emotional difficulties, and be particularly upset if an infant is impaired as a result of a technical failing during or shortly after delivery. Problems for the disabled individual concern both the technical consequences of learning to live with their illness and disability(s) and in learning and adjusting to the fact that they are different from other people. Critical stages in coming to terms with their identity occur when the child first leaves the shelter of their family on entry to school, and at the time of transition from full-time education at school. This infrequently involves further education, and may not result in entry to full-time paid work. Finally, for those individuals who are severely disabled and living in their parental home, the death of their parents may lead to institutional care.

The acquisition of a disability as a result of sudden trauma is most likely to occur among teenagers and young adults, usually as a result of accidents. The individual is likely to be initially overwhelmed by the physiological aspects and consequences of their injury. In the longer term they are confronted with the dual problem of coping with their physical losses and the restrictions of their disabilities and with coming to terms with the social disadvantages that result. Life plans and goals in the central areas of marriage, children and career may come into question or become impossible to achieve, thus posing major questions for identity and self-conception. Thus, the development of new self-conceptions incorporating their changed physical and social status is vital to successful adjustment (Morse & O'Brien 1995).

Table 7.2   Three patterns of physical disability.

Type of onset	Age at onset	Typical conditions	Main typical problems and difficulties
At birth or infancy	0–5	Cystic fibrosis Spina bifida Down's syndrome	*For parents* Shock Loss of a 'normal child' Interpreting developmental delays
			For children Mastering normal developmental tasks Learning they are different Living a normal social life despite obstacles to education, work and sexual relations
Sudden and unexpected	Teenage and young adult	Paraplegia	Shock and loss Impact on identity and self-image Rehabilitation Reconstructing their lives despite difficulties for work, leisure and sexual relations
	Middle age	Coronary heart attack	Shock Changing pattern of work and family roles and responsibilities
	Old age	Stroke	Shock Rehabilitation Dependence upon others
Slow and gradually worsening	Middle and old age	Arthritis Respiratory diseases Parkinson's disease	Maintaining a balance between normal social activities and the demands and restrictions of the condition Increasing dependence upon others For some conditions, uncertainty over stability and deterioration of condition

Other relatively common causes of sudden disability are stroke and heart attack, conditions that mainly affect the middle-aged and elderly. Although older people will experience problems of adjustment they may have fewer difficulties in adjusting to their losses and changed identities than young people. This is because they will largely have achieved (or failed to achieve) their life plans and goals.

The most common source of physical disability is long-term disease. In such circumstances the onset of disease may be slow and insidious, with a gradual process of accommodation and adjustment to increasing levels of impairment and activity restriction. This pattern is typically found in middle and, especially, old age. Increasing levels of disability as a result of the progression of a chronic illness may be one of the factors leading to retirement from paid work. At this stage of life, illness and disability may be accepted as a normal part of ageing, and psychological adjustment to them may in some respects be easier. However, there may be a greater likelihood of social isolation and people in old age may have fewer physical and financial resources to call upon in coping with their condition.

Visibility of the condition

The visibility and intrusiveness of a condition (e.g. facial burns, constant hand tremors) are important because people who are notably different in appearance or behaviour from normal expectations are most likely to be noticed. This may undermine the taken-for-granted assumptions which underpin everyday social encounters. Although chronic illness and disability are by no means inevitably stigmatising, people with highly visible impairments or disabilities are likely to experience stigmatisation (Chapter 2; Goffman 1990). Where the stigmatised condition is very visible or intrusive it may be difficult for people to escape the coercive power of attributed identities, or to have control in managing their interactions with others. They are, to use Goffman's terms, 'discredited'. At the extreme, a negative spiral of exclusion from meaningful interaction, self-withdrawal, and diminished self-esteem may result (Figure 7.1).

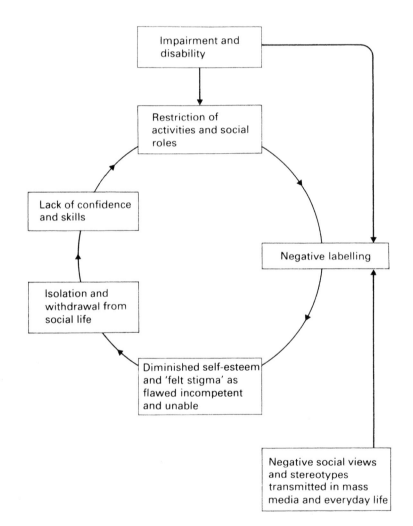

Fig. 7.1 Feedback between stigmatisation, self-esteem and participation in social activities.

With a very visible condition what many physically disabled people find very frustrating is the failure by others to recognise any aspect of their public identity other than their disability, thus failing to acknowledge all the other aspects of the person (e.g. their humour, intellectual attainment) that make up their individuality. For example, for a person with a wheelchair meeting someone for the first time, their wheelchair may provoke ideas about dependency, and feelings of sympathy and possibly embarrassment. The challenge is to move interaction on from these initial responses to engage with the interests, likes, achievement and abilities of the person with the disability. Some disability activists advocate and adopt an 'in your face' approach designed to upset normal interaction, so that others cannot feign apparent polite disinterest in the wheelchair and the disability, suggesting that this shifts the advantage to the person in the wheelchair to the discomfort of the 'normals' with whom they are interacting.

The management of interpersonal relations of a 'discreditable' chronic illness or disability whose outward appearance is not immediately apparent at the start of interaction is different. Here the disability or illness may only become apparent as interaction unfolds and as relationships develop. There are several examples reported in the literature. In the case of epilepsy, people who have that disease or members of their families may go to great lengths to conceal their illness because of their fear of the social consequences of the disclosure. This might include the loss of job, the destruction of a romantic relationship or just the loss of credibility (Scambler 1989). As noted in Chapter 2, their sense of 'felt stigma' may cause them more anxiety and distress than the actual results of disclosure and may have damaging consequences for their self-conception. Another example is people who have had ileostomies following surgery for diseases of the lower gastrointestinal tract. When they are dressed, including in swimming costumes, the ileostomy is neither visible nor obvious. However, when trying to buy life insurance, or applying for a new job the ileostomy will need to be disclosed. If they enter into a sexual relationship the ileostomy will need not just to be disclosed, but the presence of the bag and its potential to leak during sexual intercourse will need to be actively managed not just by the person with the ileostomy but also by their new partner (Kelly 1991).

While in some chronic illnesses the dominant public identity defined by the illness can be manipulated by subtle social manoeuvrings (and medication), in others, and in many physical disabilities, there is no easy escape from the symptoms or their visible salience. Not surprisingly, the advocates for persons with chronic illness and sociologists writing about them have tended to concentrate on the subtle and artful social skills which the person with a chronic illness develops to help manage their lives. The advocates of and for people with disabilities have tended to be more highly politicised and active in their opposition to what they experience as structures of oppression.

Disruption

One recurrent issue is the disruption engendered by chronic illness or disability (Bury 1997). Disruption takes many forms, going beyond disruption of the normal round of everyday activities that is true of all illness to some degree.

Symptoms are one obvious source of disruption in chronic illness and coping with a hostile social and physical environment is a major source of disruption in the case of physical disability. In some chronic conditions (e.g. multiple sclerosis) symptoms themselves can be highly unpredictable and the person may not know from day to day whether it will be a good or bad day or whether their symptoms will be intrusive or manageable (Robinson 1988). For example, in arthritis the sufferer may not know until they wake up whether it is a day when they will be able to get about easily, or whether they will be wracked by pain. It may not be clear whether medication will bring relief or not. This unpredictability makes any kind of medium- to long-term planning very difficult. The simple things in life are no longer simple.

The central issue is that many, perhaps all of the things that the person with the illness or disability wants and needs to do are made more difficult than they are for well or able-bodied people. Getting up and washing for someone with a spinal cord injury is a major task. For someone with colitis planning a simple journey is fraught with the danger of a sudden attack of diarrhoea. For someone with diabetes choosing when and what to eat are major issues. For someone with emphysema climbing a flight of stairs requires an enormous effort. Finding directions if someone is visually impaired, or listening to announcements at a railway station for the hearing impaired, are major difficulties. To be accomplished these everyday tasks require hard work, or assistance, or both. In addition, bio-medical therapeutic interventions designed to help may actually add to the burden of difficulties and make things even more complicated. Taking medication, attending hospital, undergoing investigative procedures and reorganising home life to accommodate physical needs and equipment, are all disruptive phenomena flowing from the illness that add to the difficulties the person has to cope with.

Long-term life plans are likely to become problematic, and the ideas that people have about themselves have to be readjusted. For example, someone who planned to visit Australia to see their married daughter after they had retired finds that planning such a trip is simply unrealistic. Even the notion that there will be a period of time into the future to enjoy old age may need to be significantly rethought and they are confronted with the possibility that the things they had hoped for in old age will not happen or will be significantly curtailed. As Bury (1997) puts it, biographies are disrupted in the present and into the future (this means reassessing one's past life also, so very often biographies in the past are also disrupted). Thus the individual needs to 'routinise' such disruption through the permanent rearrangement of their life if they are to achieve desired goals and maintain their quality of life.

Coping with a chronic illness or physical disability

The ways that individuals cope with their illness reflect both the stage of their condition and their personal and home circumstances at that time. People cope in a range of sometimes contradictory ways, and the ability to be flexible is vital in managing chronic illness or physical disability. As noted earlier, their material resources are also significant. A number of 'tasks' or problems in coping with chronic illness and disability can be identified. Kelly (1992) suggests that these can be considered at four levels: the technical and practical management of the condition, managing relationships with others, the management of thoughts and feelings (emotional coping), and interpreting and making sense of the condition. In one form or another these constitute the routines that make life possible and shape the ways in which identity and self will develop. Nurses may play important technical and/or supportive roles for each of these tasks.

Technical tasks

The technical tasks of coping with chronic illness and disability involve both the learning and mastery of new skills (e.g. using an artificial limb, changing colostomy bags) and gaining useful information (e.g. about how to manage special diets). These physical tasks of body management may be overlaid and infused with cognitive and emotional meaning. The technical tasks of recovery and rehabilitation may be adversely affected until these psychological, cognitive and emotional tasks have been managed. Some of these tasks, such as taking medication or the self-administration of blood or urine tests are additional to normal daily activities like dressing, eating and going to the toilet. For some people who are ill or disabled the latter may require considerable effort and/or help from others. In many conditions they have to be planned and organised in ways that can come to dominate the waking hours of the ill person and their lay carer(s).

Unless and until these technical tasks are managed successfully other aspects of life are attenuated. Physical aspects of the environment, such as ease of access to and within buildings and to transport are significant here as they enhance or restrict the lives of individuals who have a physical disability or chronic illness. Nurses can play an important role in providing information about and access to ways of improving their patients' physical environments.

Relating to others

The meanings of chronic illness and disability are not merely personal, but are the result of shared experiences and interactions with other people so another important task is that of relating to others. This may involve establishing new types of relationships with people (e.g. those involving greater dependency) and the renegotiation of existing relationships, especially within the household. These link very closely to the technical tasks described above, since the degree to which the technical difficulties posed by the condition are brought under control have a defining effect on the success or otherwise of the management of interpersonal matters.

Managing thoughts and feelings

Strong feelings and emotions may be aroused as people try to come to terms with their loss of previous abilities and social roles. People with chronic illnesses and disabilities respond with the entire range of human emotions, including anger, resentment, good humour, fear, stoicism, anxiety and depression. Such feelings can and do have a significant impact on the relationships people have with others, and both the person with the condition and those they spend time with must somehow come to live with these emotions and feelings. One response, especially following traumatic physical disability, is *denial*. This concept has come to embrace any kind of psychological response that seems to amount to failing to face up to the 'reality' of a situation. However, influenced by studies of bereavement, it is now acknowledged that denial, especially in the immediate aftermath of a trauma, can be a functionally useful response that may allow other processes of adjustment to occur (Lazarus 1985). Denial is only a problem if it persists and stops someone adjusting to their condition. *Anger* is another common response, often manifesting itself against the illness, oneself or others who are providing care. *Resignation*, giving up and submitting to an invalid status, letting their condition dominate their lives and becoming completely enveloped by the sick role is another extreme psychological response.

It is important not to see such psychological responses as inevitably pathological. Ordinary people facing extra-ordinary situations respond in extreme ways and their psychological suffering and emotional responses are likely to be highly charged. For the majority of chronically ill and physically disabled persons their emotional responses are well within the range of normal behaviour. To ignore such feelings or to view them as another form of illness is unhelpful, although there will be some persons who respond to their situation in ways that will require clinical help. Nurses may be able to help their patients and their lay carers to understand, discuss and manage their emotions by acknowledging that it is quite natural to respond from time to time with emotions such as anger or depression and that the expression of such feelings may be psychologically healthy.

Making sense of the condition

The sick or disabled person needs to be able to make some sort of sense of their condition before they can fully adjust to it. Until they can do this they may be unable to develop stable and predictable ways of managing their disability or illness. Language and storytelling play an important role here. The language used to describe the illness and its symptoms is highly important in shaping the way that people make sense of their illness (Kelly & Dickinson 1997). Among the most powerful systems in this regard is the language of medicine both through its apparent explanations of cause, treatment and outcome and through its influence on wider lay understandings of illness. However, medicine defines illness as an essentially temporary disruption of the state of health that can be restored by medical intervention, a view that does not fit easily with the realities of chronic illness or long-term physical disability.

The narratives (or stories) that people tell to others provide one of the critical mechanisms for making sense of chronic illness and physical disability (Bury 2001). Narratives about chronic illness and physical disability address long-term disruption to normal bodily and social functioning by attempting to link past, present and future in ways that establish new or reshaped identities and self-conceptions. For example, in a frequently cited paper Williams (1984) analyses how three people with rheumatoid arthritis made sense of their condition by re-constructing key aspects of their past lives (a toxic workplace, the stresses of being a wife and mother, the working of God's will). He suggests that 'narrative reconstruction is an attempt to reconstitute and repair ruptures between body, self, and world by linking-up and interpreting different aspects of biography in order to realign present and past and self with society'.

The narratives that people produce will be shaped by their own personal biographies and life circumstances, by their cultural background and beliefs, and by the type of condition affecting them, including the current point in its progression. They will vary through time, reflecting changing circumstances. In narratives the past may (indeed must) be re-interpreted in order to make sense of the present, and particular aspects of the present emphasised as being important for the future. This may involve redefining ideas what is 'good' and 'bad' in such a way as to emphasise the positive aspects of life – 'I now know who my friends are', 'I can still get out and about', 'our marriage is stronger' – and to diminish the negative consequences of illness and disability.

Bury (2001) suggests that there are three main types or levels of illness narrative. *Contingent narratives* are concerned with the origins and temporal development of the condition and its everyday effects upon the individual and others. *Moral narratives* address and sometimes attempt to shape the types of evaluative judgements that are made about people with a chronic illness and/or disability. Such narratives are essentially about changing identities and their location in social circumstance, addressing issues such as who or what is to blame and the presentation and maintenance of the person's social worth. *Core narratives* link the person's experiences with cultural meanings of illness and suffering and draw upon these shared understandings to cope with their condition, e.g. to distance oneself from the illness by using humour (Kelly & Dickinson 1997). These three narrative types perform different functions, and any story of illness or disability may include more than one of them. It is important for nurses to listen to the stories that their patients tell as this will help them to recognise important non-clinical social and psychological concerns, expectations and areas of help.

The role of others

In a very real sense the experiences of chronic illness and disability are socially defined in interaction with other people. Chapter 2 discussed the crucial role of emotional, instrumental and informational social support in illness and disability and observed that there may be some negative consequences for those providing social support. People with disabilities may challenge our ideas about what is 'normal' behaviour, possibly making us uncomfortable about the range of activities and capacities we take for granted. They may take longer over mundane tasks such as eating or dressing, may only be able to perform them in unusual ways, or require assistance with them. Not only do chronic illness and physical disability affect the individual's own activities and abilities but they may also limit the lives of other people by restricting their activities and requiring the reorganisation of their previous routines, roles and ways of viewing the world. In the short term, such disruption may be acceptable but over the long term it is likely to create difficulties for 'lay carers' and others closely associated with people with disabilities. We can identify five different types of people with whom people who are chronically ill and physically disabled have dealings.

'Normals'

The first category are those people with whom they have only casual or passing contact. 'Normals', as Goffman (1990) calls them, are likely to know very little about the condition. At this level, avoidance and stigmatisation may occur because people are ignorant, embarrassed or frightened. They may also simply be unwilling to deal with the perceived restrictions of interacting with people who have a chronic illness or disability.

Family and close friends

Close others, such as family and friends, make up one category of what Goffman refers to as 'wise' people and are the main providers of emotional and instrumental support. They have insight into the experiences of people who are chronically ill or have a physical disability because of their close association with them. The impact of chronic illness and disability upon family and friends can be profound, with their work and social life being disrupted by the needs of care and the restrictions on activity which arise from living with someone who has a disability. Close associates may themselves become stigmatised (a 'courtesy stigma') because of their relation to the ill or disabled person. Although strong emotional strains may arise, for example as a result of the burden of care or the difficulties of giving non-disabled children the care and attention they deserve, there is no evidence of higher than average marital break-up or difficulties. Research suggests that for most family carers their care is a 'labour of love' which they do willingly.

Professionals

Professional health and social workers are another important category of 'wise' people. They are in a position to shape the experience of chronic illness and disability through the instrumental help and informational support they provide, and by the way they define such illness and disability. Because of their central role in the care of people who have a chronic illness and/or disability in hospitals and the community, nurses are a particularly important group of 'wise' people. In many cases their attitudes towards the chronic illness or disability (as well as to the person who has it) may be critical in shaping the response of their patients towards it.

Chronic illnesses may be difficult for nurses to deal with because their patients won't get better and are likely to become progressively worse. In particular they may experience difficulties when they are unable to provide adequate relief of symptoms. Another difficult situation is when they are required to give 'bad news', which may lead them to pretend that there is still uncertainty about the prognosis (even though they know that there is nothing they can do or that the patient will get worse) or to disclose only some of the bad information initially, hoping that the patient will come to realise that all is not well. Nurses can provide both practical and emotional support which may enhance both the patient's coping skills and their sense of self-esteem. The provision of information and advice can be very important. Nurses can answer many questions which patients and their lay carers have about:

- The nature of their condition ('will it get worse?' 'why is the skin like that?')
- Probable activity restrictions ('will I be able to go back to work?' 'how long before we can resume sexual relations?')
- How to manage the condition ('when is the best time to do the injections?' 'I don't want to use my nebuliser too often')
- Where to find help and support ('where can I get a better bed?' 'how do I get help at night?')

They may also be able to point out the unanticipated potential for activity which may remain ('you may find that you can continue with your gardening provided that directly you feel breathless you take deep breaths and don't become anxious').

There are, however, a number of potential pitfalls. Nurses may be unresponsive to the wishes of patients and their carers because they apply their own (professionally based) judgements of need and value rather than those of the patient. Thus, they may mis-define or ignore what patients feel they need, while giving care and treatment that is perceived as inappropriate or unnecessary. What may be trivial to the nurse may be central to the patient, and vice versa. Nurses may fail to recognise the ability and knowledge that sick and disabled people and their families have about their condition and its consequences for everyday life. Because of patients' long-term involvement with their condition, perhaps including their involvement with self-help groups or other activists, they accumulate a great deal of knowledge, experience and practical wisdom about it and how best to manage it. Yet despite the increasing recognition of the important role of patient expertise in the management of their chronic illness (DoH 2001) it can be difficult to get doctors and nurses to see beyond the clinical problem to the person with wants and needs which are much broader than the bio-medical imperatives of the illness or disability. Disability activists claim that the various health and welfare institutions of British society that are intended to help them are in fact sources of their handicap and oppression (e.g. Oliver 1996). Unless nurses (and other professionals) pay sufficient attention to the knowledge and abilities of people who have a chronic illness or disability they are in danger of underestimating their abilities and preventing them being used.

Nurses, especially community nurses, may become caught up in problems associated with the frequent lack of co-ordination among care givers, and may even become caught in the crossfire of competition between different professional experts involved. Unless these various pitfalls are avoided the nurse may deliver non-responsive and even coercive advice, 'help' and care.

Alternative healers

The use of alternative healers (i.e. those with non-medical training or qualifications) by chronically ill people may in part be related to the better communication and information they are thought to provide (Sharma 1995). The main reason why people use alternative therapies is the failure of medicine to deal with chronic illness, especially musculoskeletal conditions, in a satisfactory way (Sharma 1995). Not only may modern medicine be unable to cure chronic disease, but it may also be unable to palliate symptoms such as chronic back pain adequately. Further, many sufferers find their drug therapy undesirable or the medical regimes over-invasive. The impersonality and lack of adequate information characteristic of much modern medical and nursing practice (especially in hospitals) is in sharp contrast to the time, information and personal attention received from alternative therapists. Sharma suggests that patients feel empowered and informed by alternative therapists, with greater control over the choice of treatment. Referring back to Table 2.2 (page 38), we could characterise such client–practitioner relationships as those involving guidance and co-operation and mutual participation.

Self help groups

People who may be particularly important are those with similar or the same conditions to the chronically ill or disabled person, whom Goffman (1990) calls the 'own'. The role of self-help organisations and informal contact with like situated individuals cannot be underestimated. At the personal level, self-help groups can provide mutual help and support and may be particularly important in sustaining positive self-concepts in the face of negative experiences. They can provide invaluable psychological support, insight into the person's problems and difficulties, relevant and practical information and help, and a source of sociability. At the local level they may be a valuable source of information about how to access services and can also act as pressure groups to bring about improvements. At the national level organisations such as MIND and the Disability Alliance have played an important role in raising public awareness of issues and exerting political pressure. At all these levels involvement with others with similar experiences may empower individuals to take greater control of their lives. Access to self-help and other disease-specific organisations via the internet has provided an important additional source of information and support for people with chronic illnesses and disabilities that transcends the limitations of physical proximity.

Summary

In this chapter we have focused upon fundamentally important social aspects of chronic illness and disability that cannot be subsumed within the framework of the bio-medical model. Chronic illness and disability are socially patterned, especially by age and socio-economic status, reflecting the inequalities in health manifested in society as a whole. Chronic illness and disability affect not simply bodily functioning and appearance but also self-conceptions, identities and social attachments and relationships with others. Their impact on these is influenced by the onset of the condition, its visibility and its salience for others and its disruption of everyday life. Four key tasks were identified in coping with a chronic illness or physical disability: the technical and practical management of the condition; managing relationships with others; emotional coping; and interpreting and making sense of the condition. Finally, other people, including nurses, have an important role in shaping the experience of chronic illness and disability.

References

Bone, M. & Meltzer, H. (1989) *The Prevalence of Disability among Children.* Office of Population Censuses and Surveys/HMSO, London.

Bunker, J. (2001) *Medicine Matters After All: Measuring the benefits of medical care, a healthy lifestyle, and a just social environment.* The Stationery Office/Nuffield Trust, London.

Bury, M. (1997) *Health and Illness in a Changing Society.* Routledge, London.

Bury, M. (2001) Illness narratives: fact or fiction? *Sociology of Health and Illness,* **23**, 263–85.

Charmaz, K. (1983) Loss of self: A fundamental form of suffering of the chronically ill. *Sociology of Health and Illness,* **5**, 168–95.

Darling, R. (1979) *Families Against Society: A Study of Reactions to Children with Birth Defects.* Sage, New York and London.

Davey, B. & Seale, C. (eds) (2002) *Experiencing and Explaining Disease* (3rd edn). Open University Press, Buckingham.

DoH (Department of Health) (2001) *The Expert Patient: A New Approach to Chronic Disease Management for the 21st Century.* The Stationery Office, London.

Goffman, E. (1990) *Stigma: Notes on the Management of Spoiled Identity.* Penguin, Harmondsworth.

Kelly, M.P. (1991) Coping with an ileostomy. *Social Science and Medicine,* **33**, 115–25.

Kelly, M.P. (1992) *Colitis.* Routledge, London.

Kelly, M.P. & Dickinson, H. (1997) The narrative self in autobiographical accounts of illness. *Sociological Review,* **45**, 254–78.

Kelly, M.P. & Field, D. (1996) Medical sociology, chronic illness and the body. *Sociology of Health and Illness,* **18**, 241–57.

Lazarus, R.S. (1985) The costs and benefits of denial. In: *Stress and Coping: An Anthology* (eds A. Monat & R. Lazarus). Columbia University Press, New York.

Lupton, D. & Seymour, W. (2000) Technology, selfhood and physical disability. *Social Science and Medicine,* **50**, 1857–62.

Matheson, J. & Summerfield, C. (eds) (2000) *Social Focus on Young People.* The Stationery Office, London.

Millward, L.M., Morgan, A., & Kelly, M.P. (2003) *Prevention and Reduction of Accidental Injury Evidence Briefing.* Health Development Agency, London. www.hda-online.org.uk/evidence

Morse, J.M. & O'Brien, B. (1995) Preserving self: from victim, to patient, to disabled person. *Journal of Advanced Nursing,* **21**, 886–96.

Oliver, M. (1996) *Understanding Disability: From Theory to Practice.* Macmillan, Basingstoke.

Priestly, M. (1999) *Disability, Politics and Community Care.* Jessica Kingsley, London.

Robinson, I. (1988) *Multiple Sclerosis.* Routledge, London.

Scambler, G. (1989) *Epilepsy.* Routledge, London.

Sharma, U. (1995) *Complementary medicine today. Practitioners and Patients,* revised edn. Routledge, London.

Strauss, A.L., Corbin, J., Fagerhaugh, S., Glaser, B.G., Maines, D., Suczek, B. & Weiner, C.L. (1984) *Chronic Illness and the Quality of Life,* 2nd edn. Mosby, St Louis.

Wanless, D. (2001) *Securing our Future Health: Taking a Long Term View: Interim Report.* HM Treasury, London.

Williams, G. (1984) The genesis of chronic illness: narrative reconstruction. *Sociology of Health and Illness,* **6**, 175–200.

Further reading

Barnes, C., Mercer, G. & Shakespear, T. (1999) *Exploring Disability: A sociological introduction.* Polity Press, Cambridge.

Davey, B. & Seale C. (eds) (2002) *Experiencing and Explaining Disease,* 3rd edn. Open University Press, Buckingham.

Chapter 8
Mental Disorders

In any social situation there are expectations as to how people should normally behave and communicate. At one time those whose behaviour departed radically from social norms were variously labelled as 'idiots', 'lunatics' or sometimes as 'possessed' by demons or evil spirits. However, in modern societies it is generally accepted that such people are suffering from mental disorders and in need of care and treatment from specialist health professionals. To many people this trend is an indication of a more enlightened, humane and compassionate society. Others disagree, arguing that many mental disorders are not 'really' diseases and to label them as such may be counterproductive by further restricting the opportunities of the mentally disordered to live comparatively normal lives and, sometimes, legitimising an oppressive form of social control over them.

This chapter will:

- Compare different theoretical approaches to mental disorders
- Look at changing patterns of care of the mentally disordered
- Examine suicidal and self-harming behaviour
- Consider the relationship between psychiatric care and social control

Approaches to mental disorders

The term mental disorder covers a wide and ill-defined area, but it is possible to distinguish between three overlapping populations. First, there are those suffering from impaired bodily function, such as people with learning disabilities or senile mental confusion. Second, there are people with behavioural problems, such as eating disorders or alcohol or drug abuse, who are often treated by health care professionals *as if* they had diseases. Third, there are those who have what are called mental illnesses, such as schizophrenia or depression, and there is considerable debate here about whether such conditions are diseases or behavioural problems.

There are many different theoretical approaches to mental disorders, but abroad distinction can be made between biological, psychological and sociological perspectives (Table 8.1). Biological theories argue that all, or most, mental disorders are symptomatic of an underlying *bodily* malfunction and offer, and occasionally impose, medical treatments of one sort or another. Psychological theories suggest

Table 8.1   Models of mental illness.

	Medical	Psychological	Social
Definition/ diagnosis	Mental illnesses are diagnosed by doctors in terms of clearly defined criteria and are symptoms of underlying *bodily* disease.	Mental illnesses are diagnosed by doctors or therapists. Precise diagnosis difficult. Mental illnesses are diseases of the *mind* which may, or may not, have an organic basis.	Diagnosis of mental illness problematic. Often owes more to social factors than clinical evidence. Behaviour 'labelled' as 'illness' may be response to difficult, or oppressive situation.
Causes	Uncertain, but growing evidence of genetic predisposition and biochemical causes.	Often caused by experiences in patients' past, especially in early childhood.	Triggered by social circumstances that create stress, lower self-esteem and sense of control.
Treatment	Medical, surgical and nursing care.	Psychoanalysis to help reveal subconscious conflicts or cognitive disorder. Behaviour modification.	Individuals may require help and treatment in short run, but condition will not improve if changes are not also made in their life situation.
Goal	To restore patient to health through treatment, or at least control symptoms and prevent condition getting worse.	To give patient insight into origins of problems and help develop strategies for combating them.	To help reduce rates of mental illness by revealing social influences.

that some mental illnesses and behavioural disorders may be a product of personal experiences that distort thought processes and are thus 'diseases of the *mind*' rather than the body. Psychological theories do not necessarily reject biological influences or medical treatments, but argue that they should be accompanied, or substituted, by various therapies aimed at giving people more insight into the psychological sources of their mental distress or behavioural disorder. Sociological approaches focus on *relationships* between individual experiences of mental disorder and distress and wider patterns of social organisation. Sociologists are interested in the role of social influences in the *causes* of mental disorder, its *recognition* and the organisation of treatment and care of the mentally disordered.

Biological approaches

Many mental disorders (such as Down's syndrome) or mental confusion (such as Alzheimer's disease) are now known to have organic bases. However, with mental illnesses, evidence of biological causation is far less conclusive. Mental illnesses are typically divided into psychoses and neuroses although, in practice, it is sometimes difficult to distinguish between them. In general terms, psychotic states involve a distorted perception of reality and can sometimes be very frightening for the sufferer, relatives and nurses. In contrast, sufferers from neurotic disorders, such as obsessional compulsive behaviour, usually have insight into their problems and seek treatment.

Schizophrenia is a generic name for a group of psychotic disorders that tend to manifest themselves in early adulthood. Schizophrenic behaviour is characterised by disordered thought patterns, a loss of touch with reality, hallucinations, and may include trances and rigid body postures (catatonic schizophrenia) and fears of persecution (paranoid schizophrenia). It has long been believed that schizophrenia is a disease of the brain and technological advances, such as magnetic resonance imaging (MRI), have revealed abnormalities in the brain of *some* schizophrenics, giving new momentum to the old idea that some mental illnesses, particularly psychotic conditions, are diseases.

Types of mental illnesses tend to run in families, which suggests a genetic predisposition to the disease, but in practice it is difficult to isolate genetic influences from environmental ones. Biological research has also suggested that mental illnesses may be the result of imbalance of chemicals in the brain called neurotransmitters. For example, there is some evidence that schizophrenia may be the result of over-activity of the neurotransmitter called dopamine, while depression and self-harming behaviour have been linked to low levels of another neurotransmitter called serotonin. In this context, treatment involves trying to correct the imbalance with medication. However, there are difficulties with this bio-chemical approach. First, the results of studies have been inconsistent. Secondly, even if research did reveal a consistent association between brain chemistry and mental illness, it would be difficult for researchers to be sure whether they were discovering cause or effect, as biochemical changes in the brain might be a *consequence* of stressful life experiences. It is thus also important to take into account the influence of external events in triggering mental illnesses.

Psychological approaches

Most psychological theories focus on neuroses and behavioural disorders, and attempt to locate the sources of the disorder in the patient's experiences. A number of theories have examined the relationship between the 'formative' experiences of early childhood – especially traumatic experiences – and mental disorder in later life. Psychoanalytical theory argues that there are crucial stages in the *emotional* development of the child, such as separation from the mother and the recognition of sexual identity. Unresolved conflicts at one or more of these crucial stages can remain in the person's *unconscious* mind and produce anxieties and neuroses in later life. Psychoanalytic therapy aims to help to provide insights into the childhood origins of the patient's present distress. While many feel they have benefited from such therapy, its clinical effectiveness remains unproven, as it is difficult to test objectively.

Cognitive psychology focuses on thought processes in the *conscious* mind and argues that there are distinct stages in the child's *intellectual* development as it comes to think rationally about itself and the world. From this perspective, it is argued that factors (such as traumatic childhood experiences) can impede this process and lead to distorted cognitive perceptions in later life. For example, the stage of cognitive development where the child starts to appreciate the effect of its actions on others may fail to materialise for various reasons, leading to a 'psycho-pathic' personality where acts of gross cruelty can be undertaken without any apparent remorse. In cognitive psychology, thought processes are seen as causal influences in their own right and not mere reflections of bio-chemical changes or unconscious impulses. Cognitive therapy therefore focuses directly on the patient's 'irrational' or 'distorted' beliefs, testing them against reality and trying to establish more rational perceptions.

Other, more social psychological, approaches try to locate the sources of mental disorder in *social* relationships, particularly within the family. In a classical study developing this 'family model', Laing and Esterson (1964) attempted to show that 'schizophrenic' behaviours were in fact unconscious 'strategies' to cope with unliveable family situations. From this point of view, the source of mental illness is the *interaction* between the patient and other family members. Schizophrenia is evidence of a disordered family rather than simply a disordered individual. This approach has been widely criticised as unscientific and untestable, as well as failing to explain why people exposed to more or less similar experiences do not also become schizophrenic. However, the 'family model' of mental illness has been influential and many practitioners treating mental disorders focus on families rather than individuals. More recent research in this area has explored the role of families in the *course* of mental illness rather than as its cause. A number of studies have suggested that the chances of relapse into mental illness amongst discharged patients is much more likely when they are returned to families with high levels of expressed emotion, such as hostility, criticism and over-concern (Lopez *et al.* 1999). From this perspective, it is argued that rehabilitation programmes need to focus on patterns of interaction in families, particularly the management of expressed emotion.

Sociological approaches

Despite the important differences between, and within, biological and psycho-logical approaches, there are also similarities. Both tend to work within established medical definitions of mental disorder and both attempt to locate its causes within the bodies, or minds (or both) of individuals. The sociological critique of this 'medical model' of mental disorder is that it tends to ignore the social contexts from which mental disorders emerge and are recognised and treated. Two distinct sociological approaches can be identified. The first explores the extent to which recognised psychiatric conditions, such as anxiety or depression, are caused by social factors. The second is more concerned with the *social reaction* to mental disorders, and to mental illness in particular.

Social causes

Epidemiological research has shown that specific mental disorders, such as schizophrenia and depression, are not distributed randomly in populations but are consistently linked to socio-demographic variables, suggesting that mental dis-orders may also be caused by factors in the wider social environment. For example, rates of recorded mental disorders for people from Afro-Caribbean groups and for some groups of Asians are higher than for the general population (Chapter 3). Women have higher rates of reported mental disorder than men, although men are slightly more vulnerable to schizophrenia (Chapter 4). Mental disorders appear to be more common in urban areas and most – but not all – research studies have found that rates of mental illness are higher amongst the lower social classes, or socially deprived (Gomm 1996; Weich *et al.* 2001).

Although socio-demographic factors are positively correlated with mental disorders, they are not in themselves causes. Research involves trying to explain *why* factors, such as low social class, are associated with mental disorder, how they are linked to other factors and why particular individuals within these groups are more vulnerable. Brown and Harris' research into the social origins of depression provides a seminal example of this approach (Brown and Harris 1978, 1989).

Brown and Harris were interested in identifying the differing life situations and associated stress factors that led to higher rates of depression amongst working-class women compared to middle-class women. Working-class women were doubly disadvantaged. First, they were more likely to experience long-term major life difficulties, such as poor housing and financial problems, and major stressful life events, such as death of a family member or unemployment. Second, they were more *vulnerable* to the effects of stress (Chapter 2). This was because certain key 'vulnerability factors' – the presence of three or more dependent children at home, the loss of a mother before the age of 11, lack of paid employment and absence of a close confiding relationship – were all more common amongst working-class women. These factors had the effect of lowering self-esteem and making women more vulnerable to the damaging effects of stressful life events. As they arose from *social* situations, Brown and Harris concluded that although depressive illness is a biological condition, its origins lay in social factors.

Social reaction to mental disorders

While the sociological approach described above explores how social factors may contribute to the onset of biological mental disorder, other sociologists have adopted a more sceptical approach and questioned the diagnostic categories themselves, particularly in relation to mental illness. They are interested in why some actions (but not others) are seen as symptoms of mental illness and why some individuals (but not others) are labelled as mentally ill. For example, as we saw in Chapter 4, some researchers have argued that the higher rates of mental disorder in Britain found in people of Afro-Caribbean origin, are the result of differential diagnostic processes.

One of the most influential sociological works in this *societal reaction* tradition is that of Scheff (1966). He argued being 'mentally ill' is a social role, the entry to which owes less to the nature of the symptoms themselves than to the reactions of others to them. When people's behaviour *regularly* fails to meet expectations of others, *and* where other explanations of their behaviour fail, they are likely to become labelled as 'mentally ill'. Such labelling is influenced by factors such as the amount, visibility and intrusiveness of the symptoms. Family and friends will tend to accommodate, and even deny, very strange behaviour for long periods before they reluctantly resort to defining their partners or relatives as mentally ill. Thus, the tolerance of other people is an important factor. Different types of behaviour seem to be tolerated more readily in some groups than in others, for example, schizophrenic behaviour in manual working groups. Other factors include the relative power and status of the person (more powerful and high status persons are more able to resist the label), and whether other roles are available, such as the witch doctor or shaman in some pre-industrial societies, or the eccentric or tortured genius in modern society.

A key role is played by stereotypes of madness that are learned in early childhood and reinforced by the mass media and in ordinary social activities. In the crisis surrounding labelling the stereotypes of madness clarify and make sense of the strange and unpredictable behaviour. While it appears that stereotypes of the mentally ill as bizarre, dangerous and unpredictable, are being complemented by more accepting and less stigmatising ideas about less severe mental disorders, research by Philo *et al.* (1996) found the media images were still more likely than not to demean and stigmatise mental illness, with two thirds of all such items linking mental illness and violence. In the process of 'making sense' of mental illness in everyday life, a person's past behaviour may be selectively reconstructed, and signs of individuality and previously acceptable idiosyncrasy become reinterpreted as signs of incipient madness. Professional health workers, including psychiatric nurses, are also prone to reinterpret a person's behaviour in terms of their label of mental illness (Rosenhan 1973). People who become labelled as mentally ill also know the common stereotypes, and may come to accept their applicability to themselves and incorporate them into their self-conceptions and behaviour. Once they have been defined as mentally ill they are 'rewarded' for playing the role of the mentally ill – that is, doing what doctors and nurses want them to do – and 'sanctioned' for not doing so. Treatment regimes may lead to a great loss of independence and individuality, especially in hospital settings, and non-compliance may lead to 'punishments' in the form of further curtailments of activity.

The societal reaction approach has been criticised on a number of grounds. First, it is seen as being more applicable to the comparatively rare psychotic disorders than to the more common neurotic disorders. Secondly, critics argue it underplays the extent to which individuals may willingly embrace the sick role, allowing them legitimately to give up the struggle to live a normal life. Third, it does not explain the origins of mental disorder, only the reactions to it. However, in spite of these limitations, the societal reaction approach makes a valuable contribution to understanding some forms of mental disorder. It draws attention to the problematic nature of psychiatric diagnoses and the fact that – in part at least – the behaviour of those labelled as mentally ill may be a consequence of being socialised into a 'mentally ill role'.

Care of the mentally disordered

In modern societies the delivery of care to people with mental disorders continues to be organised primarily around psychiatric diagnoses and interventions. This is most evident in the hospitalisation of those with mental disorders but, even in the community, psychiatric and medical definitions constrain and influence the behaviour of other health workers, social workers, lay carers and, as we have seen, the mentally disordered themselves. The following sections consider hospital and community care separately although, in practice, many people with mental disorders regularly move to and fro between hospital and community.

Hospital care

Once defined as mentally ill a person may be treated by their GP or as an outpatient at a psychiatric unit attached to a general hospital. Most psychiatric hospital care is now delivered in acute psychiatric units of general hospitals, often in a series of short admissions and discharges. When a person is severely disturbed and considered to be a risk to themselves or others, they may be compulsorily admitted to a hospital and they can, if deemed necessary, be treated without their consent. The vast majority of mental health admissions are voluntary, but research has shown that a significant minority of 'voluntary' patients have either been threatened with compulsory admission or feel that they have been coerced into hospital (Pilgrim and Rogers 1999).

Within psychiatric hospitals, where many patients are disorientated and incapable of giving consent to their care and treatment, hospital staff, particularly nurses, exert great influence upon patient behaviour. Recovery prospects are influenced both through the way that nurses interact with patients and through their definitions of them (Prior 1993). A major criticism of institutional care – supported by some well-publicised scandals and official inquiries – is that staff in mental hospitals are more likely to abuse their powers and compromise patients' rights. However, these criticisms have to be put into context as there are a number of important differences between psychiatric mental health nursing and general nursing. First, while the majority of patients with mental disorders are not aggressive or threatening, staff in mental hospitals, and psychiatric wards, do run a higher risk of being assaulted than staff in a general hospital. There are now around 60 000 reported assaults against NHS staff each year and the majority take place in mental health settings. Second, psychiatric services have traditionally been under-funded and wards and institutions characterised by low staffing levels, high demand for physical care and many confused residents are more likely to produce a vicious circle of neglect, lack of stimulation and low staff morale. Third, mental health nursing gives rise to specific practical and ethical difficulties, particularly where patients have to be treated without their consent or restrained for their own safety or the safety of others. For example, staff have to make difficult decisions about the extent to which medication should be used purely to restrain patients, or whether or not secluding troublesome patients is justified (Griffiths 2001).

Sociological studies of mental hospitals have been less concerned with the real or alleged failings of health workers than with the impact of the organisation of the hospital on both professional practices and the course of the patient's illness and their sense of identity. For example, in a highly influential study, Goffman (1991) argued that admission to a mental hospital may result in what he called a 'mortification' of the patient's self-concept. The restrictions on movement, the need to fit into the on-going routines of hospital, having to ask permission for, or help with, things previously taken for granted can erode the patient's self-esteem and sense of autonomy. In some cases this results in a state of childlike dependency that could then be interpreted by nurses as *further* evidence of mental illness and psychological deterioration. A particular danger for chronically ill psychiatric patients is that they might become so used to long-term hospital care that they become 'institutionalised' and unable to function in the community. Indeed, the confusion and apathy often found amongst patients in mental hospitals and residential homes, may be the result of long-term institutional care and excessive medication, rather than mental disorder.

Growing realisation that the structure and organisation of mental hospitals was essentially pathogenic led to a number of reforms from the 1950s, with more mental hospitals developing 'open door' policies, workshops and half-way houses. One of the most radical reforms was the development of 'therapeutic communities' in the 1960s and 1970s, where hospital routines were made more flexible and egalitarian and attempts were made to break down some of the hierarchical divisions between staff and patients. The 'group' became a therapeutic tool, decisions were made collectively and patients were encouraged to create their own treatments, often by redefining everyday events as part of therapeutic work. However, as mental hospitals began to contract and close and the pressure on existing beds increased, many of these reforms were abandoned and mental hospitals slowly reverted to the 'warehouses' they had been in the first half of the twentieth century.

De-institutionalisation

Between 1950 and 1990, the number of residents in mental hospitals in England and Wales fell from almost 150 000 to under 50 000. During the 1990s the numbers continued to fall, but much more slowly and there was an increase in numbers in 2001 (Table 8.2).

Table 8.2 Number of residents of mental hospitals in England and Wales, 1990–2000*. Crown copyright.

1991	48700
1992	45100
1993	39500
1994	36400
1995	34800
1996	34550
1997	34550
1998	31750
1999	30800
2000	29900
2001	31500

*Estimated by unfinished patient episodes
Source Department of Health.

There are many reasons for the declining number of residents in mental hospitals in the second part of the twentieth century. First, successive governments, confronted by the escalating costs of health care, came to favour care in the community as a cheaper option. However, economic factors alone cannot explain de-institutionalisation, as it was well underway before the major economic crises in health care in 1970s and 1980s. A second factor was a 'pharmacological revolution' (Le Fanu 1999). The development of psychoactive drugs in the 1950s, particularly chlorpromazine, helped control the symptoms of many psychotic conditions enabling more patients to function outside hospital. Thirdly, the cumulative weight of evidence about the negative aspects of long-term institutional care contributed to the movement towards community care.

It is important to appreciate the wider social significance of de-institutionalisation. The asylum represented a clear division between the sane and the insane, with the latter locked safely away. With de-institutionalisation, the boundaries between sanity and insanity, or mental disorder and mental health, became blurred. On the one hand, there was some de-medicalisation as many of those previously seen as insane were redefined as people with various 'difficulties', and in need of social care in the community. On the other hand, there was a medicalisation, or more specifically a 'psychiatricisation', of everyday life as psychiatrists, looking for a new professional focus, uncovered widespread and untreated mental health problems in the community. In the last two decades the American Psychiatric Association has 'discovered' (critics would say invented) almost 200 new mental syndromes, including 'frotteurism' (touching others on public transport) and 'fugue' (travelling under an assumed identity) and 'generalised anxiety disorder' (Kutchins and Kirk 1997). In short, in contemporary mental health thinking, few are really mad, but comparatively few are in good mental health. Mental disorder (insanity) and mental health (sanity) are two poles of a continuum, with the majority of people located somewhere in-between.

Community care

There are many definitions of community care but, in general terms, it means non-institutional care. It is important to realise that community care is not a value-neutral term. It describes a set of principles and policy initiatives that the majority of people involved in health care feel are desirable and worthwhile. Arising from the dissatisfaction with institutional care, the idea behind community care is to give people with mental (and physical) disorders greater autonomy and self-determination by enabling them to live in the community and, as far as possible, make choices about their own lives. The 'care' aspect involves providing assistance in developing their skills, enhancing their self-respect and maximising their participation in everyday activities. However, community care does not just refer to a set of policies, it *also* describes the organisation and delivery of non-institutional care in the real world. It is therefore important to distinguish between community care in principle and community care in *practice*.

The principles of community care

The first and most basic principle of community care is providing suitable accommodation for those leaving mental hospitals. This involves support for people who
return to live with their own families, and developing facilities for those who do not,
ranging from highly staffed 'hostel wards' and group homes, through shared
accommodation with some professional support, to single-person flats with minimal
support.

A second key principle is 'normalising' mental disorders as far as possible. This
was originally developed with reference to people with 'mental handicap', now
called learning disabilities, and later extended to other aspects of mental health
where medical intervention, particularly biologically based approaches, had little or
no tangible benefit. Normalisation strategies aim to enhance cognitive and social
skills and promote ordinary life in three main ways by providing:

- Positive role models
- A range of practical instruction and skill enhancement activities, and
- Greater integration of people with mental disorders into the community

This involves developing more places of support within the community, such as day
care centres, and modifying social and physical environments in order to preserve
or enhance functioning in spite of continuing disabilities. However, despite the
laudable aims behind normalisation, ex-patients who are insufficiently independent
should not be left to make choices and decisions of which they are incapable. It is,
therefore, very important that community nurses make a careful assessment of
what can, and cannot, be realistically achieved by a client.

A third key principle of community care, stemming from normalisation, is that of
'de-medicalising', as well as de-institutionalising, more aspects of mental disorder.
This involves a transfer of responsibility of the care of more people with mental
disorders from the NHS to local authorities (Chapter 11). Professional intervention,
from being the exclusive concern of health care professionals, became a multi-
disciplinary responsibility, with nursing, social services and other relevant local
agencies offering 'frontline' social and primary health care, such as health education, casework with long-term chronic cases and 'crisis management', including
organisation of psychiatric referrals in acute cases. More recently, this approach
has been developed further with the development of *inter*-disciplinary 'community
health teams' that aim to provide a more comprehensive and integrated service.

The practice of community care

Research has suggested that there are large gaps between the aims of community
care and their realisation in practice. A major criticism is that the development of
suitable accommodation in the community has not kept pace with the numbers of
people leaving mental hospitals. Former mental patients are more likely than the
general population to be living in group accommodation or on their own or be
homeless (Brandon 1991). Some ex-mental patients are cared for by their families.

While some families cope willingly and effectively, others experience great difficulties. Manifestations of mental disorder such as confused speech, muteness or unpredictability may be disruptive, upsetting and difficult to cope with. Families may also be more indirectly affected through the stigma they acquire, or feel they acquire, because of their relationship with the ex-patient. They may also have to cope with their own feelings of shame, guilt and anxiety. Family members may thus try to hide the fact of the ex-patient's hospitalisation, and distance themselves from them in various ways. They may also be affected economically by having to give up, or reduce, their paid employment. Despite the introduction of a Carers (Recognition and Services) Act 1995 designed to address some of these problems, there is little evidence to suggest that the situation is changing significantly (Tee & Dorey 2000).

The success of 'normalisation' strategies and the community care of the mentally disordered, people with learning disabilities and others whose behaviour is unacceptable or difficult to relate to, depends upon their genuine integration into everyday social life. Their mere presence in a community does not equate to their *integration* into that community. The evidence is not encouraging. Discharge from hospital is often accompanied by (justifiable) fears about negative attitudes and discrimination and social exclusion in the community (Sayce 1999). Such attitudes contribute to the difficulty of setting up 'half-way houses' and other community-based treatment schemes for people with mental disorders. The idea that such conditions are essentially incurable persists, and so ex-mental patients may be avoided and find it difficult to resume their previous work and family roles. It is thus not surprising that a common strategy followed by ex-mental patients is that of 'passing' for normal by hiding the fact of their hospitalisation and diagnosis from others. Community care requires more than government action and good health care, it also requires fundamental changes in social attitudes. It is very important that those working with people who have, or have had, mental disorders do not unintentionally 'conspire' with these negative views by underestimating their clients' abilities and potential skills.

While an integrated approach to community care makes sense in principle, it has been difficult to achieve in practice. In organisational terms, it has often been difficult to co-ordinate the work of health and social services and determine the responsibilities of each sector (Rogers and Pilgrim 2001). There are also problems in delivering community mental health initiatives. Research has shown that community mental health teams, for example, are characterised by poor planning, random case allocation, inter-agency conflict and poor communication (Chalk 1999).

Although institutional care and community care are often seen as alternatives with the latter increasingly replacing the former, it is also important to appreciate how they linked in practice. As a result of the diminishing number of hospital beds, a large number of acutely mentally people are either not admitted to hospital or discharged very quickly after admission. This means that an increasing number of community mental health workers then have to spend more of their time managing emergency cases at the expense of their primary and long-term case-work. The irony of this is that community mental health teams, specifically set up as an *alternative* to institutional care, have become a major route back into hospitals.

Re-institutionalisation?

The movement from institutional to community care should not be exaggerated. First, while the numbers of psychiatric in-patients in Britain has declined sharply since 1955, NHS hospitals remain a major place of treatment, and the estimates of the number of residents in mental hospitals actually rose from 29 900 in 2000 to 31 550 in 2001 (Table 8.2). Secondly, rates of admission to mental hospitals have risen and patient throughput has more than doubled in the past ten years, with many hospitals stretched to breaking point and exceeding their 100% occupancy rates. It is now common for many mental patients to be discharged only to return to hospital after a short time in the community in a 'revolving door' pattern of care. Around 70% of hospital admissions are now re-admissions (Turner *et al.* 1999). Third, a consequence of the depopulation of long-stay mental hospitals has been a growth in the institutional care of the mentally disordered in prisons and in the private sector (Simpson 2000). In short, not only are many mental patients still treated in hospitals, many others have simply been moved from one form of institutional care to another. With mental hospitals now so overcrowded, criticisms of lack of care in the community and increasing public fears about the dangers posed by some mentally disordered people, it is impossible to escape the conclusion that while the old asylum system institutionalised too many people, the brave new world of community care has too few hospital beds. It is a lesson governments and health policy makers are just starting to learn.

Suicide and deliberate self-harm

One of the major dangers of mental disorder and mental breakdown is the increased risk of deliberate self-harm. Each year in Britain about 6000 deaths are recorded as suicides, a rate of just over 11 per 100 000 population (Figure 8.1). Suicide is the second most common cause of death in people under twenty-five. According to official statistics, males are three and a half times more likely to kill themselves than females. However, it would be wrong to view suicide and self-harm as a predominantly male problem. Females are more than twice as likely to attempt suicide as males and certain forms of chronic self-harm, such as eating disorders and self-mutilation are much more common in women. It is also significant that, while the suicide rate of older women has fallen significantly, there has been little change in the rate of younger women. As Pritchard (1995) observes, 'in every region of Britain, younger women are dying significantly more often from suicide than other women'. Some researchers have predicted that as women's patterns of employment come to resemble men's, their patterns of suicidal behaviour will come to resemble those of men.

  Whilst the official statistics provide a useful guide to patterns of suicidal behaviour, they are only the 'tip of an iceberg' of suicide and deliberate self-harm. Many 'suicidal' deaths are simply not recorded in the official statistics (Chapter 1) and it is generally accepted that suicide rates underestimate the true rate of suicide. Further, an estimated 150 000 people each year commit serious acts of deliberate self-harm that would have led to death without medical and nursing intervention.

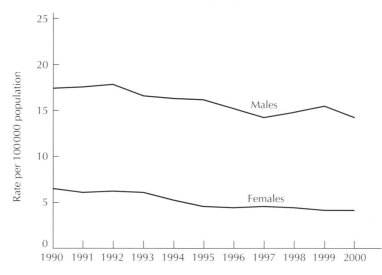

Fig. 8.1   Suicide and undetermined deaths in the United Kingdom, 1990–2000.
Source   ONS, Crown copyright.

   Research into the ways that people in modern societies go about harming themselves has contradicted some of the 'common sense' assumptions typically made about suicide. A common error that people (including doctors and nurses) make in trying to understand suicidal behaviour is to assume that a clear distinction can be made between 'genuine' suicidal acts (aimed at death) and 'false' suicidal acts (cries for help). Detailed reconstruction of the circumstances of suicidal acts has proved this assumption to be false. The majority of acts of deliberate self-harm, including many that end in death, are desperate gambles with life and death where the result is decided by factors outside the individual's control. In pioneering research, Stengel (1973) showed that most suicidal acts are not simply aimed at death and dying, but also at life, survival and contact with others. In most cases suicidal individuals give warnings of their intentions and try to communicate their unhappiness and growing despair to others. For example, most suicidal acts take place in a setting (usually the home) where others are present, and use a method (usually poisoning) where rescue is possible.
   The observation that most suicidal acts are undertaken with ambivalent intent and are preceded by attempts to communicate unhappiness and despair has implications for prevention and for nursing suicidal and potentially suicidal patients (Taylor & Gilmour 1996). Indications of possible suicidal intent may include:

- Direct warnings of suicidal inclination, which should be taken seriously
- A preoccupation with death and dying
- Expressions of worthlessness and of being a burden
- Dramatic mood swings
- Significant change in behaviour
- Giving away treasured possessions
- Calls to say goodbye to people

Understanding of these 'suicidal clues', coupled with known risk factors, such as depression, unemployment, little social support (Chapter 2) and a history of a previous attempt can help the nurse to make a reasonable assessment of suicidal risk. Partly as a result of their mistaken beliefs about the intent of people who overdose, nurses and doctors tend to be impatient with overdose patients. They are often treated harshly in casualty, ignored on the wards, and made to feel they are wasting staff time. Such reactions, although understandable, are likely to reinforce the already negative self-attitudes of suicidal patients and make a re-attempt more likely.

Suicide is a particular risk among those suffering from depressive disorders, especially those who are coming out of their depressive state. Yet, despite the association between mental disorders and suicide, the majority of those who deliberately harm themselves do not have a clinical mental illness. Most are suffering from an emotional breakdown, often triggered by some personal crisis, and have come to see suicide as the only solution. The observation that suicidal behaviour is not necessarily a symptom of psychiatric illness has implications for intervention and support. The therapy offered by doctors, psychiatrists and psychiatric nurses can be invaluable in helping to manage psychiatric conditions. However, the tendency of many people to 'medicalise' unhappiness and take their emotional problems to doctors can be counterproductive (Chapter 2). Not only are drugs unlikely to be effective in the long term, as unhappiness and emotional problems are not diseases, but there is the possibility of iatrogenic consequences, such as dependency and overdosing. Three quarters of those who overdose have seen their doctor in the two weeks before they harm themselves, and the majority use medically prescribed drugs. While medication can be helpful for people in emotional crises, a greater proportion of suicidal and potentially suicidal patients and clients need to be listened to rather than medicated. In such cases, psychological approaches may have more to offer than biological ones

Suicidal behaviour can raise a number of legal and ethical dilemmas for nurses. Attempting to commit suicide has not been illegal in Britain since The Suicide Act of 1961, but it is still a criminal offence under the Act to assist someone to commit suicide. Most ethical issues concerning suicide revolve around the contradictions that can arise from a person's autonomous right to determine their own life and the obligation on the part of health professionals to protect a person believed to be incapable of making a rational decision for themselves. The observation of patients believed to be at risk of harming themselves and others typically falls on nurses. Not only does this involve practical problems, but it can also be seen as a violation of patient rights and a contradiction of the consumerist ethos of the modern health service (Dimond 2000). However, even though some may feel it is ethically wrong to restrain a potentially suicidal patient, legally a nurse who does not take reasonable care to protect a patient known to be a suicidal risk can be sued in the civil courts for negligence.

Other less directly life-threatening self-damaging conditions, such as alcoholism and eating disorders, pose similar dilemmas about the relative autonomy of patients and responsibilities of staff. For example, the forced feeding of anorexics creates emotional and ethical problems for many nurses. These conditions also raise the question of whether such self-damaging behaviour is best viewed as a rational choice that life is no longer worth living or a symptom of a disease amenable to medical intervention.

Care or control?

Underlying the growth of psychiatric care for the mentally disordered is the assumption that many mental disorders are diseases that should be managed and treated by health care professionals. This assumption was questioned by some in the second half of the twentieth century. Most controversy surrounds the notion of mental illness. We have observed that some sociologists have argued that defining someone as mentally ill often owes more to social than to clinical considerations and that being labelled as 'mentally ill' can significantly affect a person's self-image and subsequent behaviour.

Other critics go further. Szasz (1987) argues that the very notion of mental illness is a myth. He distinguishes between physical and mental illness. Symptoms of physical illness are *objective* signs (e.g. cancerous cells), whereas the symptoms of so-called 'mental illness' are *subjective* assessments about a person's behaviour and the extent to which it deviates from socially acceptable norms. According to Szasz, while the physician makes a scientific diagnosis about a patient's body, psychiatrists and psychiatric nurses make value judgements about a patient's behaviour. He does not deny that many psychiatric patients suffer psychological distress, but argues that these people have 'problems in living' and not mental illnesses. Thus it makes little sense to offer them medical treatment, that is designed to correct deviation from biological norms. Furthermore, as long as 'mental illness' is blamed for so many of peoples' problems in living, it detracts attention from the real causes, which may lie in adverse life circumstances, moral conflicts, intolerance, or social injustices. By defining behaviour that departs from social expectations as 'illness' and offering to cure it, the psychiatric professions are helping to reinforce accepted ways of thinking and legitimising the treatment, and sometimes the compulsory detention, of those who deviate from them. From this point of view psychiatry, psychiatric nursing and mental health legislation are much more about the *social control* of people whose behaviour is causing problems for others than they are about the *care* of sick people. According to Szasz, the myth of mental illness persists in modern societies not because of its scientific validity, but because it is such an effective means of social control.

This view has been criticised both for underestimating the effectiveness of contemporary psychiatry and for overestimating its social control function. However, it does raise important ethical issues. At the core of nursing (and medical) ethics is the principle of acting in the patient's interests. The fact that many people have not chosen to be treated in mental hospitals, but are there because others, such as family members, managers of residential institutions or the courts want them there, strikes at the heart of this most fundamental principle. Practices such as the hospital treatment of alcoholics and those with eating disorders, the compulsory admission of patients, and the widespread administration of major tranquillisers, raise ethical issues that psychiatric nursing cannot avoid. However, criticism of existing psychiatric practices, particularly when they involve the curtailment of patients' rights, have to be balanced against the importance of treating people who may be in no position to give their consent and who may be a danger to themselves or to others. Should people who are unable to look after themselves be left sleeping rough on the streets? Should those refusing to eat be left to starve? Should a person expressing persistent murderous intentions towards another be left until they kill? In the last decade, in the wake of a number of well-publicised cases where former mental patients have harmed either themselves or others, there has been mounting criticism about lack of institutional care for, and control of, the mentally ill (Morrall 2000).

Simply to observe that some psychiatric care is a form of social control is to do little more than state the obvious. Most psychiatric professionals are well aware of the control elements involved in their work. The key ethical issue in this context is whether the forms of control offered by psychiatric care in hospitals, or in communities, operate for or against the interests of the mentally ill. Psychiatric care, for all its acknowledged inadequacies, has to be balanced against leaving the mentally disordered to fend for themselves or to face criminal punishment and possibly imprisonment.

Summary

Mental disorder covers a wide range of conditions from recognised diseases to behavioural problems treated as if they are diseases. Explanations of mental disorder and models of treatment are mainly based upon biological and psychological theories. Sociological research has drawn attention to the role of wider social influences on the origins and recognition of mental disorder and on the organisation of care. From the middle of the twentieth century, there was widespread criticism of the institutional care of the mentally disordered, many of whom were seen as needing social care rather than medical treatment. The numbers of people in mental hospitals declined dramatically throughout the second part of the twentieth century and more people were cared for in the community. However, not only has community care failed to live up to the expectations vested in it, but many of those with mental disorders have simply exchanged one form of institutional care for another. People with mental disorders are at much greater risk of suicide and self-harm, but many of those who harm themselves are not clinically ill and there is a risk of medical treatment doing more harm than good. Some critics have suggested that psychiatry is intellectually flawed and that psychiatric care is more about controlling people than caring for them. In this context, the crucial question is whether the 'medicalisation' of human madness and desperation tends to serve the interests of the vulnerable patient or those of wider society in controlling those it finds troublesome.

References

Brandon, D. (1991) *Innovation without Change?* Consumer Power in Psychiatric Services. Palgrave, Basingstoke.

Brown, G. & Harris, T. (1978) *Social Origins of Depression: a study of psychiatric disorder among women.* Tavistock, London.

Brown, G. & Harris, T. (eds) (1989) *Life Events and Illness.* Unwin and Hyman, London.

Chalk, A. (1999) Community mental health teams: reviewing the debate. *Mental Health Nursing*, **19**, 12–14.

Dimond, B. (2000) Confidentiality 12: the problems posed by suicide and euthanasia. *British Journal of Nursing*, **9**, 52–3.

Goffman, E. (1991) *Asylums: essays on the social situation of mental patients and other inmates.* Penguin, London.

Gomm, R. (1996) Mental Health and Inequality. In: *Mental Health Matters* (eds T. Heller, J. Renolds, R. Gomm, R. Muston & S. Pattison). Open University Press, Buckingham.

Griffiths, L. (2001) Does seclusion have a role to play in modern mental health nursing? *British Journal of Nursing*, **10**, 656–61.

Kutchins, H. & Kirk, A. (1997) *Making Us Crazy.* Free Press, New York.

Laing, R. & Esterson, A. (1964) *Sanity, Madness and the Family.* Penguin, London.

Le Fanu, J. (1999) *The Rise and Fall of Modern Medicine.* Little, Brown & Co., London.

Lopez, S., Nelson, K., Synde, K. & Mintz, J. (1999) Attributions and effective reactions of family members and course of schizophrenia. *Journal of Abnormal Psychology*, **108**, 307–14.

Morrall, P. (2000) *Madness and Murder.* Whurr, London.

Philo, G., Secker, J., Platt, S., Henderson, L., McLaughlin, G. & Burnside, J. (1996) Media images of mental distress. In: *Mental Health Matters* (eds T. Heller, J. Renolds, R. Gomm, R. Muston & S. Pattison). Open University Press, Buckingham.

Pilgrim, D. & Rogers, A. (1999) *A Sociology of Mental Health and Illness.* Open University Press, Buckingham.

Prior, L. (1993) *The Social Organisation of Mental Illness.* Sage, London.

Pritchard, C. (1995) *Suicide – the Ultimate Rejection? A psycho-social study.* Open University Press, Buckingham.

Rogers, A. & Pilgrim, D. (2001) *Mental Health Policy in Britain*, 2nd edn. Palgrave, Basingstoke.

Rosenhan, D. (1973) Being sane in insane places. *Science*, **179**, 250–58.

Sayce, L. (1999) *From Psychiatric Patient to Citizen: overcoming discrimination and social exclusion.* Palgrave, Basingstoke.

Scheff, T. (1966) *Being Mentally Ill: a sociological theory.* Aldine, Chicago.

Simpson, A. (2000) Private care's win win. *Mental Health Nursing*, **20**, 6–9.

Stengel, E. (1973) *Suicide and Attempted Suicide.* Penguin, London.

Szasz, T. (1987) *Insanity: the Idea and its Consequences.* Wiley, New York.

Taylor, S. & Gilmour, A. (1996) 'Towards understanding suicide'. In: *Mental Health Matters* (eds T. Heller, J. Renolds, R. Gomm, R. Muston & S. Pattison). Open University Press, Buckingham.

Tee, S. & Dorey, T. (2000) Families and schizophrenia. *Mental Health Nursing*, **20**, 10–13.

Turner, T., Salter, M. & Deahl, M. (1999) Mental health reform: should psychiatrists go on being responsible? *Psychiatric Bulletin*, **23**, 578–81.

Weich, S., Lewis, G. & Jenkins, S. (2001) Income inequality and the prevalence of common mental disorders in Britain. *British Journal of Psychiatry*, **178**, 222–7.

Further reading

Barnes, M. & Bowl, R. (2001) *Taking Over the Asylum: empowerment and mental health.* Palgrave, Basingstoke.

Pilgrim, D. & Rogers, A. (1999) *A Sociology of Mental Health and Illness*, 2nd edn. Open University Press, Buckingham.

Chapter 9
Death, Dying and Bereavement

Death has real and symbolic significance in our society. It generates questions about the meaning of life and how death is defined. It raises moral questions about euthanasia and end-of-life care and poses ethical dilemmas about confidentiality and the 'right to know'. All these occur in the context of an ageing, multi-cultural, society where groups have different beliefs, values and priorities in relation to death. Nurses are the main group of staff involved in the care of people who are dying in all settings of care. This chapter will focus upon one of the main determinants of the experience of dying: where dying and death occurs. It will also consider influential models of dying and bereavement, communication and awareness and end-of-life issues. However, it does not consider other important social variables such as social class, gender and ethnicity which shape not only experiences of death and bereavement, but also their likelihood (Field, Hockey & Small 1997). While people die at all ages, and miscarriage, stillbirth, and the deaths of infants and children are of concern, in this chapter we concentrate upon adults, especially at older ages, as this is when most deaths occur. The chapter will:

- Summarise the historical context of death in Britain
- Identify and discuss patterns of dying in different settings, comparing the care provided to people with cancer to those with other non-malignant conditions
- Discuss changing patterns of communication and awareness of dying
- Discuss current models of bereavement
- Discuss euthanasia and end of life care

Death in contemporary Britain

Over the course of the twentieth century dramatic changes occurred in the patterns of death and dying in Britain. In 1901 life expectancy at birth was 49 for females and 45 for males. This had increased to 80 and 75 by 2000. The main source of this was the decrease in infant mortality from 19–13% in 1901 to less than 1% at the end of the century. Life expectancy of adults increased more slowly, but by century's end over 80% of the population could expect to reach the age of 65. The length of survival beyond 65 continues to increase (Chapter 6). Acute infectious diseases have been superseded by long-term chronic conditions as the major causes of death. Whereas formerly people would experience a number of deaths among those with whom they were closely associated, in the present era children rarely experience the death of a close friend or family member, and even for adolescents and adults such deaths are uncommon (although the increasing number of deaths from AIDS has altered this among some groups). Deaths from drug and alcohol abuse among young people are increasing rapidly and suicide is now the major cause of death among those aged below 35.

Most deaths result from chronic and degenerative diseases primarily affecting middle-aged and older adults. The leading causes of death in 2000 were diseases of the circulatory system (39%), respiratory system (17%) and cancers (25%). Most of the attention to death and dying of adults in contemporary Britain has focused upon cancer, with hospice and specialist palliative care services developing in response to this. Since the 1990s there has been an increasing recognition that those (generally older) people dying from heart disease, strokes and respiratory diseases are equally in need of specialist palliative care. Entering the new century the extension of such services to these diseases is a high priority.

Another major change over the century has been the institutionalisation and 'medicalisation' of death, i.e. the shift of the normal place of death from the home to a hospital or other institution. In 2000 only 18% of deaths occurred in the person's own home and 78.5% occurred in hospitals, hospices, or nursing or residential homes (Table 9.1). Men are significantly more likely to die in their own home than women, who are more likely to die in a nursing or residential home. This is partly explained by the greater longevity of women. Relatively few people in our society die sudden and unexpected deaths. The majority of unexpected deaths of young people are caused by accidents, only a minority of which reach a hospital. Among older people, heart attacks and strokes are the main causes of sudden, unexpected death. Again, most victims die prior to entry to the hospital, and those that do may be treated in intensive or coronary care units.

Scholars such as Aries (1983) and Elias (1985) have suggested that dying and mourning have become highly individualised in modern society. As a consequence

Table 9.1 Place of death, England and Wales, 2000.

Place of death	Male	Female	All
NHS hospital	58%	55%	56%
Nursing homes	7%	13%	10%
Residential homes	4.5%	11%	8%
Hospice	4.5%	4%	4%
*All institutional**	*74.5%*	*82%*	*78.5%*
Own home	22%	15%	18%
Other*	3.5%	2%	3%
Number of deaths	255 547	280 117	535 664

*Includes non-NHS psychiatric hospitals.
Percentages do not sum to 100 due to rounding.
Source National Statistics (2002) Mortality Statistics, General Review of the Registrar General on Death in England and Wales 2000. Stationery Office, London. Calculated from Table 17.

of the reduced immediacy of death and the decline of religion there are few of the collective family and community rituals that in previous eras made sense of death and supported the bereaved. Thus, when they are faced with coping with their own death or that of someone close to them people may have to come to terms with this unfamiliar event without the help of clear collective rules, and with little support from the wider community. Sontag (1989) suggested that diseases such as cancer are particularly feared, and act as metaphors for more general and widespread anxieties about dying and death. The 'medicalisation' of dying has provided one source for making sense of death, dying and grieving in our society, although doctors and nurses may themselves have difficulty coping with the wider questions about the meaning of death. Another source of 'meaning making' may be the plethora of media stories and autobiographical accounts (usually about cancer) that provide 'templates' for how to manage a 'good dying' and 'appropriate mourning'. Although death is no longer a 'taboo' subject in contemporary Britain, it remains largely hidden and 'sequestered' from public view (Mellor 1993; Walter 1994). The solution for many people is to place the onus for dealing with death and dying upon doctors and nurses.

The main settings of care

The focus of this section is the places where dying occurs. This is not necessarily the same place as where people die: whilst less than a third of deaths occur in the places where people live, the majority of their care takes place in these domestic and care homes. There may be a lot of interchange between home, hospital and hospice with the involvement of a wide range of hospital, community and specialist palliative care services over the course of an advanced condition. The co-ordination of these various lay, statutory, voluntary, and commercial sources of help (Fig. 9.1) to provide 'joined up' or 'seamless' care for those who are dying has been recognised by the Government in its National Service Frameworks as central to effective end-of-life care.

Dying in a hospital

NHS hospitals are the major sites of death in our society. Most of these deaths are of adults beyond middle life. The shift towards community care (Chapters 8, 10) has meant that hospitals are increasingly becoming places of acute, intensive, short-stay treatment with long-term care being managed in the community (including residential and nursing homes). Hospital specialist staff (including nurses) working with patients with chronic advanced conditions are likely to be involved in the management of their care in the community. In contemporary Britain circulatory diseases account for two fifths of all hospital deaths, cancers for a fifth, and respiratory diseases just under a fifth. A significant number of deaths in hospitals occur over a relatively short period of time and death is a rare occurrence in many hospital settings.

Our understanding of dying in hospitals is largely based upon studies of cancer

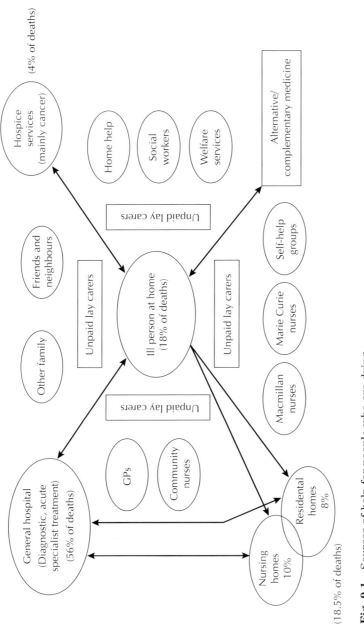

Fig. 9.1 Sources of help for people who are dying.

Source Field, D. & James, N. (1993) Where and how people die. In: *The Future for Palliative Care* (ed by D. Clark). Open University Press, Milton Keynes. Reproduced by permission Open University Press.

settings where dying took place over a long period of time and death was anticipated by the staff, and sometimes by patients. However, Field's (1989) research
concerned non-cancer patients and Seymour (2001) discusses the management of
death and dying in intensive care. Many of the insights from the early studies of
cancer deaths are still valid. For example, the *time* over which death occurs and its
predictability are still major factors affecting how staff experience terminal illness
and treat dying patients (Glaser & Strauss 1965). In general, hospital staff have most
difficulty in dealing with quick and unexpected deaths and are most comfortable
with deaths which are predictable and which can be prepared for. Another
important factor is the *age* of the patient. In our society people find it is easier to
accept the death of old people than of young people. In particular nurses find it
psychologically difficult to nurse infants and young children who are terminally ill,
and people of their own age with whom they may identify such as those with cancer
or AIDS. Finally, as discussed below, communication and disclosure of information
are central to the care of dying patients.

A number of developments, especially in more effective and reliable pain and
symptom control, more widespread understanding of the benefits of palliative care
and the introduction of specialist palliative care teams have improved the care of
dying hospital patients, although this still seems to vary widely both within and
between hospitals. The number of staff involved in such care has increased, and the
co-ordination of the various elements of the treatment of terminal conditions has
become more complex. This means that the interdisciplinary co-ordination of care
is important. Nurses, who are at the centre of care delivery, may thus be confronted
with delicate and difficult tasks of negotiating potentially conflicting treatments and
'do not resuscitate' orders with doctors and others. Because of their continuous and
close contact with the dying patient, nurses may become aware of the need for a
shift to palliative care before doctors. It seems that it is still often difficult for the
latter to move from therapeutic, and possibly aggressive, management of disease
towards a pattern of care where other needs of patients and their quality of life are
seen as primary.

The continuing development of technology and knowledge has led to sophisticated
interventions into matters of living and dying, and demands on nursing staff continue
to increase (Chapter 12). This may raise questions of skill mix and responsibility and
cause difficulties in delivering patient-centred care in accordance with the body of
knowledge and expertise which nursing has developed. Changes in working patterns
also affect the emotional involvement that develops between nurses and patients,
perhaps making these more transitory and less intense. Yet, given the nature of
nursing work, emotional involvement with some patients, especially long-term
patients in specialist units, is likely to develop, with a sense of loss when the patient
dies. While nursing a dying person may be stressful, Vachon's (1995) review of the
evidence suggests that the main source of such stresses was the work environment.

Care in the home

About 90% of the care of people who die will take place in their own homes with the
help and unpaid work of their close family and friends ('lay' carers, see Chapter 10).

People who die at home will normally do so as the result of a long-term illness, often marked by persistent and distressing symptoms. It is thus highly likely that at some time they will have been admitted to a hospital or (in cases of cancer) a hospice for treatment of their condition. The evidence is that most people would prefer to be cared for and to die in their own home. For example, Hinton (1994) found that in the week before their death 54% of the terminally ill patients he interviewed said they preferred to be cared for at home, although less than half (45%) of their spouses held that view.

The desirability and possibility of a 'home death' depends primarily on the human resources available to help both patients and carers and, as Hinton (1994) observed, carers may have different needs and attitudes to the dying person. For the dying person the main advantages are that the familiar environment can provide psychological comfort, reassurance and support. They are also more likely to be able to retain greater autonomy and control of what happens to them than in an institution, at least during the time they retain mobility and mental clarity. For their lay carers, caring can be rewarding, maintaining and perhaps reinforcing family ties. However, the physical and social costs of caring for those caring on their own or with little outside help may be substantial, making their care work tiring and even a burden. Although many carers wish to look after their relative at home, a range of factors may make this difficult or impossible. The two main problems for home care are the adequate control of symptoms and the constant attendance and extra domestic work that such care entails. Failure in either or both of these will lead to institutional care. Some carers (and patients) feel that a home death would make it difficult for them to continue living in their home following the death. It has been suggested that lay carers will cope better with their bereavement if they can take an active part in care, and this is easier at home than in a formal institution.

Changes in population and social structure mean that there are now more people without family or relatives to provide unpaid home care than in previous times (Chapter 10). Older women are particularly likely to be affected by this. The physical help and social support given by general practitioners and community nurses and their access to other resources of help is thus vital. Having an outsider to talk to and to ask advice from can help lay carers keep a sense of perspective. A community nurse may also be very important in negotiating in-patient care when it is necessary and in helping lay carers to come to terms with the fact they can no longer manage on their own. On-going and recently completed but unpublished research (in 2002) suggests that support in the home is significantly better for those dying from cancer and their carers than for those dying from chronic non-malignant conditions. In part this reflects the higher priority given to people with cancer. In part it reflects the difficulty that doctors have in recognising when dying is imminent for people where the continuing benefits of therapeutic admissions to hospital may persist until the admission during which the patient dies (Field 1998).

Hospice care

Hospice care originally focused around in-patient centres of excellence promoting holistic care of dying people in a homely environment. Since the mid-1960s, when there were only a few mainly in-patient units, hospice and specialist palliative care services have expanded dramatically and now take a variety of forms (Table 9.2). The volume of patients treated has remained largely unchanged since the mid-1990s. For 2002, the Hospice Information Service reported 58 000 hospice admissions and 1200 patients seen by home care teams. Hospice services are mainly offered to cancer patients (96%) but people with other conditions such as motor neurone disease may also be referred to them. People from minority ethnic groups are under-represented among users of hospice and specialist palliative care services, a matter of concern (Firth 2001).

Table 9.2 Hospice and palliative care services in the UK and Ireland, 2002.

*Voluntary units (2443 beds)	217
NHS units (596 beds)	56
Children's hospices (186 beds)	25
Day care services	243
Home care services	334
'Hospice at home'	78
Hospital support teams	221
Hospital support nurses	100

* Includes three services (64 beds) exclusively for HIV/AIDS
Source A. Jackson & A. Eve (eds) (2002) *Hospice Services and Palliative Care Services in the United Kingdom and the Republic of Ireland.* St Christopher's Hospice Information Service.

Referral to a hospice or specialist palliative care service is an important signal that an illness is regarded as 'terminal', conveying the message that death, if not imminent, is not too far away. This may lead to discussions with the person who is dying about their concerns and wishes. Talking about the person's death and dying is expected to be one of the strengths of hospice staff and is central to addressing psychological, social and spiritual aspects of dying as well as attending to physical symptoms. The hospice approach to such holistic care is to encourage the expression of all forms of pain so that they may be attended to. Thus, the nurse's role in supporting the patient is based on an understanding of the patient's emotions and not simply a narrow focus upon their physical pain. This inevitably leads to some emotional involvement with patients and those close to them and although attachments occur these are more likely to be seen as rewarding than as a source of distress. Important components of coping with the inevitable deaths of patients are staff support and 'permission to grieve', (which may be denied to nurses in other settings). The supportive environment of the hospices and their focus on agreed goals of care should mean that there are fewer major difficulties of workplace stress than elsewhere (Vachon 1995).

The nature of referral as an in-patient to hospices has changed significantly, with many patients admitted for short-term symptom management. Continuing symptom appraisal and management may occur as part of hospice day care visits. An important result of this changing pattern of in-patient admission is that the length of time that patients stay in hospices has reduced significantly, but that re-admissions are more common. Another significant change is that the proportion of in-patients with difficult-to-manage and distressing symptoms has increased. One such group are patients with bodies that are disfigured, seeping fluids or unpleasant smells: what Lawton (2000) describes as 'unbounded bodies'. She describes how such patients move from being socially valued individuals to increasingly isolated objects of self-disgust as their bodily disintegration leads to their social and physical separation from others and their withdrawal from social interaction. Nursing such 'dirty' dying patients is a challenge to the hospice philosophy of enabling patients to live until they die with all their needs attended to, and challenges the ability to achieve the desired 'good' and dignified death. Although it is likely that at the time of her research in 1998 the hospice she studied was atypical, the shifting case mix within hospices suggests that such situations will become more common, thus posing increasing challenges for nurses working in hospices.

Dying in an institutional care home

Nursing and residential homes have become increasingly important locations for the care of old people who are dying. Changes in the NHS since the 1990s have meant that nursing homes have largely replaced long-stay hospital wards for longer-term symptom management and nursing care. Greater numbers of dying people are now admitted to nursing homes from NHS hospitals than previously and in-patient hospices are also referring patients for admission to nursing homes. At the turn of the century some 18% of deaths occurred in these settings (Table 9.1).

In their discussion (upon which this section draws) Field and Froggatt (2003) point out that most people living in institutional homes are there either because they have no-one to care for them at home or because such carers are unable to continue to do so. The new elderly resident often sees entry into the care home as the final move of their life. The challenge for care homes is to provide both supportive care for their 'fit' and 'frail' residents and end-of-life care for those approaching death. Perhaps the most fundamental challenge here is the pattern of morbidity and the nature of dying found in care homes. Residents in such homes as compared to those living in their own homes or those of relatives are more likely to:

- Be suffering from chronic and long-term conditions
- Have significantly greater restrictions of their activities
- Have higher levels of mental confusion
- Have higher levels of incontinence, impaired sight and hearing

It is often difficult for staff to identify those who are dying. The majority of residents who die do so from chronic conditions other than cancer are likely to have multiple clinical conditions, often persisting for many years. Thus there is often a great deal of uncertainty about whether or not residents are actually dying. For example, 42% of the deaths in one large-scale study were the result of 'general deterioration' (51% in nursing homes) and only 9% from an already recognised terminal illness (Katz & Peace, 2003). In these circumstances it may be difficult for residents to become involved in decisions about how their end-of-life care should be managed.

Care homes typically have very limited resources to manage end-of-life care and the quality of such care is thus greatly influenced by external services. Only in nursing homes will there be trained nursing staff and health care assistants. The low level of trained staff means that it may be difficult to manage the needs of residents living with on-going chronic conditions and adds to the difficulties caused by the disease profile of residents for recognising, and meeting, their needs for end-of-life care. Thus the contributions – or lack of them – from external sources significantly influence the care of dying residents. General Practitioners and community nurses play a vital role in the care of residents in nursing and residential homes. For example, General Practitioners are the primary resource for pain control and referral to palliative care services. However, where home staff are trained for end-of-life care, but General Practitioners are not, conflicts can occur, for example, over pain management. Admission from care homes to hospitals is less likely to occur than from domestic homes. When hospitals (and hospices) transfer patients with advanced diseases to nursing homes this may occur so close to death that it is inappropriate. Few care homes use hospice and specialist palliative care services. Although local hospices are potential sources for the management of difficult symptoms and for terminal care, access to them may be difficult for care home residents, particularly those with conditions other than cancer.

In many homes acknowledgement of death and dying is not overt. In part this may reflect negative societal attitudes towards older people (Chapter 6). Where death is accepted and integrated with living (e.g. in homes run by religious organisations), staff, residents and relatives may be able to talk openly about forthcoming events, including the possibility of dying. In such homes the bereavement needs of other residents are also more likely to be appreciated and attended to.

Dying and bereavement

In contemporary Britain the education of nurses and others working with dying and bereaved people has been based primarily upon psychodynamic, individual-centred understandings of grief and loss, although it is recognised that social dimensions such as age, gender, community affiliation and social attachment, shape and influence individual responses to bereavement (Field, Hockey & Small 1997; Payne, Horn & Relf 1999).

Dying and bereavement have both personal and social aspects: not only are personal attachments lost, but so are social relationships, connections and activities. Further, the experiences of dying and grieving, both before and after the death, are greatly affected by social and physical circumstances such as where dying and death takes place, the types of communication between those involved, and the social support available. For example, both the dying person and their partner will lose their relationship to each other and the shared social activities which they participated in as a couple. Attachment to others is a source of emotional and psychological strength and support, and a source of social cohesion (Chapter 2).

But it is also a source of pain, loss and distress when attachments are under threat or severed.

Dying

The work of Kubler-Ross (1970) alerted those working with dying hospital patients to the need to take account of the psychological reactions which dying people experience. She proposed that a number of stages could be identified in the psychological adjustment of hospitalised cancer patients to the knowledge that they were dying (denial, anger, bargaining and acceptance). Despite the positive impact of Kubler-Ross's ideas in focusing nursing attention upon the isolation and psychological difficulties of dying patients, her work has been criticised. Although the emotions she describes may be found in dying patients, they vary from person to person and not everyone experiences all of them and oscillation between different emotional states is normal. There is danger in taking Kubler-Ross's work as prescriptive, rather than as a guide to what might be expected, for example interpreting anger as a positive sign that the patient is 'making progress', while neglecting to pay adequate attention to possible remediable causes of such anger (e.g. unrelieved pain). Attempts may be made to 'move' the patient on 'to the next stage' and some nurses may feel that they have failed if their patient dies without reaching 'acceptance'. Further, extreme adherence to the Kubler-Ross approach leads to excessive expectations of what nurses and doctors can do, while devaluing the wishes and abilities of the dying person to cope with their dying and death in their own way. The idea that nurses can solve all the social and psychological problems which dying patients have, can make death pleasant, and can overcome years of family ill-feeling is unrealistic. While retaining the important message that the patient's psychological reactions vary and must be attended to, it is also important to be aware of both the great variability in the way people respond to dying and the important role of social circumstances in shaping these.

Bereavement

In hospitals the main focus of nursing work and concern with dying people is with specific individuals, with little sustained provision (or capacity) to care for the grief and mourning of relatives and friends. These are more likely to be the province of General Practitioners and community nurses, although the research evidence suggests that most bereaved people have no sustained contact with professional carers.

'Traditional' models typically portray bereavement as a process during which the grieving individual passes through a number of phases or stages over a period of time (Payne, Horn & Relf 1999). 'Normal' reactions to bereavement have been described as occurring in approximately sequential but overlapping phases of grief lasting about two years, although there are differences between people in terms of both the duration and form of each phase (Parkes 1996). It is suggested that typically the initial shock, disbelief and 'numbness' following the death may last from a few hours to a week. This is often followed by a chaotic period characterised by anger, distress, restlessness, and 'searching' for the lost person. Denial may also occur. In this period of acute grief, the bereaved person may vacillate between seeking reminders of the dead person to assuage their sense of loss and avoiding them in order to escape from their grief. Familiar places, activities and sounds may all vividly recall the dead person, and many people report talking with, hearing or seeing the dead person. This is seen as a crucial stage where the reality of the death becomes confirmed and accepted. The bereaved person may experience a number of physical symptoms, such as weight loss and sleep disturbance. This period is followed by a time marked by disorganisation and sometimes despair as the person comes to grips with their various losses and changes of activities, begins to learn new skills, and develops new patterns of living. Finally, it is proposed, a stable pattern of life may achieved when the person has resolved the problem of retaining their connection with the dead person while 'letting them go' and continuing with their own life. Individuals may become 'stuck' or move 'backwards' and 'forwards' between stages and emotions may fluctuate over time. Using this generic model, suggests that the 'work' or 'tasks' of grief involve a process of 'letting go' of the dead person in order to return to normal social and psychological functioning (Worden 1992).

The dual-process model (Stroebe & Shut 1999; Figure 9.2) moves beyond the view of bereavement as a generally unilinear progression of the individual through time, stressing oscillation between 'loss orientation' (focusing on the deceased and the death, confronting and dwelling on their loss) and 'restoration orientation' (the practical tasks of adjusting to a new pattern of life). Both of these aspects must be dealt with, and healthy adaptation is a dynamic process involving both expressing and controlling emotions and dealing with concurrent life changes. At times their

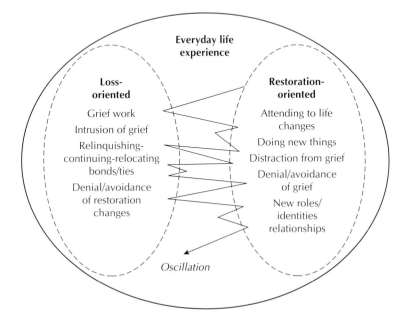

Fig. 9.2 The dual-process of grief. Reproduced with permission from Margaret Stroebe and Henk Shut.

demands can be so overwhelming that people may need to take 'time out' from
them. Both 'loss' and 'restoration' related behaviours are important in coming to
terms with bereavement and will vary according to gender, social and cultural
background and personal circumstances. By moving the focus of explanation away
from loss, the dual-process model directs attention to the variety of emotional and
practical 'coping tasks' involved in adjustment to bereavement. However, despite
the acknowledged role played by social factors, the focus remains firmly upon the
individual.

During the 1990s sociological analysis of how grief is shaped by the social contexts and relationships of the bereaved has strengthened our understanding of the
centrality of the social dimensions of bereavement. The work by Riches and
Dawson (2000) on parental and sibling responses to the death of a child shows how
parents draw upon social networks and cultural ideas to make sense of and adapt to
their grief. It also integrates existing evidence with their own research to show how
the different socially patterned responses of men ('stoic' control of emotions, focus
upon practical tasks) and women (expressing emotion) to their loss may create
strains between partners. Walter (1999) uses the work of Durkheim (Chapter 1) to
discuss 'the integration of the dead and the living', and the regulation or 'policing' of
grief. He draws upon anthropological and contemporary material to support his
analysis of the variety of ways that bereaved people reshape their relationships with
those who have died. In doing so he challenges some basic assumptions of 'traditional' stage/phase conceptualisations of grief, especially the assumption that grief
is 'resolved' by 'moving on' from and 'letting go of' one's connection with the person
who has died. On the contrary, many people want to 'hold on' to and remember
those who have died and continue to include them in their lives in a variety of ways
(Klass *et al.* 1996). To do so does not mean that they have somehow 'failed' to
resolve their grief, or are grieving 'pathologically'. Walter emphasises that talking to
others about the deceased is an important way of establishing the meaning of
relationships and that the dead live on through such conversations. Like Riches and
Dawson, he discusses gender differences and challenges the current emphasis upon
encouraging the expression of grief and discouraging its containment. Both Riches
and Dawson and Walter draw upon their analyses to suggest practical implications
for the support and care offered by those working with the bereaved.

Secular and religious ceremonies associated with the disposal of the dead body
perform both psychological and social functions by confirming and reinforcing the
fact of death. They also serve to validate the social worth of the deceased, to
confirm the relationship of the mourners to them and to each other, and may
mobilise social support for the bereaved. These are important functions because
grieving may become complicated when the fact of death is uncertain or denied, e.g.
when there is no body, and social isolation and lack of support are associated with
difficulties with grieving. Elaborate rituals extending over a period of time can be
found in some communities. These may serve to limit and guide mourning and to
shape social support by providing a structure in which there is a gradual tapering off
of the connection of the bereaved with the dead person.

Recent research and anecdotal evidence suggests that despite the significant
developments in understanding grief and bereavement outlined above, most health

workers and counsellors continue to work with implicit 'stage/phase' models that see bereavement as something to be 'worked through' to guide their understanding of bereavement and their work with bereaved people who need their help. It is important that nurses are aware of these new developments and that they become integrated into their practice, for example by 'allowing' the bereaved to maintain their continuing bonds with the deceased.

Communication and disclosure

The seminal work of Glaser and Strauss (1965) identified four types of 'awareness context' which have profound consequences for the experiences of dying patients. These were:

- *Closed awareness*, where staff kept patients in ignorance of their impending death, usually with the co-operation and agreement of their relatives
- *Suspicion awareness*, where patients suspected that they were dying and tried to get staff and relatives to confirm this suspicion
- *Mutual pretence*, where all parties knew that the patient was dying but did not acknowledge this, pretending that 'everything was normal'
- *Open awareness*, where all parties knew about and acknowledged that the patient was dying

They found that 'closed awareness' contexts were preferred by staff for a number of reasons including their uncertainty about when death might occur and to 'protect' patients from adverse psychological reactions to disclosure, such as depression and anxiety. Closed awareness also allowed hospital staff and relatives to avoid the emotionally difficult task of talking about the terminal diagnosis and its meaning for the patient. However, they found that closed awareness was hard to sustain and that it tended to 'break down' and become transformed into 'suspicion' or 'mutual pretence'. Their work, and that of other researchers, suggested a number of negative consequences of the closed awareness context for patients such as the physical and social withdrawal of staff and relatives from the patient, isolation, loneliness, increased uncertainty and anxiety, and a sense of betrayal resulting from the restricted information and communication about their condition and its progression. Open awareness contexts, by contrast, were thought to prevent or resolve these negative consequences, to enable more informed and more effective management of pain and other symptoms and to facilitate patient acceptance of, and preparation for, their death. This is a distinctly 'anglophone' perspective. In other cultures (e.g. Italy and Japan) closed awareness is seen as protecting the dying person from distress and many groups within culturally diverse societies such as Britain and the USA will share this view (Turner 2002).

In practice, 'open awareness' appears to be ambiguous and conditional, with patients at one moment recognising, acknowledging and preparing for their death and at a subsequent time apparently denying that they are dying. Copp and Field

(2002) suggest that 'denial' and 'acceptance' of dying may be used by patients within the overall context of open awareness as strategies to avoid threats and to preserve existing relationships. Timmermans (1994) argues that reactions vary within and between patients and distinguishes three types of open awareness. In *suspended open awareness*, the patient (and/or relative) 'blocks out the information provided about the terminal condition'. This may be a temporary, initial, reaction to the shocking information, or it may persist. Suspended open awareness may reappear in situations where unexpected decline or improvement occur. In this awareness context, although the information has been given, the tacit understanding is that the patient's impending death will not be discussed or publicly acknowledged. *Uncertain open awareness* results from the tendency of doctors to control the information given to patients by withholding, softening or otherwise modifying the 'clinical truth' about prognosis. A key element is the attempt by doctors and nurses to use uncertainty about outcome to maintain a 'margin for hope'. *Active open awareness*, as in Glaser and Strauss's concept, is where all parties understand and accept that recovery from the impending death is not possible and try to come to terms with this.

Despite the evidence that in contemporary Britain both health workers and the general public prefer the management of dying in an open awareness context this is often difficult to achieve, especially in long-term non-malignant conditions where uncertainty about the likely time of death may persist and where timing the move from an essentially 'curative/restorative' focus of treatment to 'palliative care' may be difficult to determine (Field 1998). Many nurses and doctors find the task of actually transmitting this information very difficult and stressful, and few have received adequate training in appropriate communication skills. When nurses are uncomfortable about talking openly with patients about their likely death – even where they believe that this is the right thing to do – it is likely that they will avoid or limit their contact with them to a greater or lesser extent. This is especially likely to occur where death is uncommon, where there is little team support to nurses, and where there is no clearly formulated policy regarding disclosure. Researchers have found that in their day-to-day encounters with dying patients health workers moderate and back away from automatic disclosure of a terminal prognosis (Field & Copp 1999). Reasons given for withholding or modifying the information given to terminally ill patients are:

- The patient's level of comprehension
- The stage of the illness
- The mental competence of patients
- The severity of illness
- To maintain hope
- Moral scruples

Field and Copp (1999) suggest that a pragmatic and responsive pattern of communication and disclosure that recognises the rights of patients to full information and open awareness, whilst acknowledging that not all patients will want this, seems appropriate. This may be particularly important with patients from some cultural and religious backgrounds. However, one danger of adopting this approach is that nurses and doctors might not provide opportunities for patients to discuss their dying thus preventing them from voicing their wishes and needs, which may remain unrecognised or misunderstood and unmet. Nurses must balance the advantages of openness and the respect for the emotional, cultural and informational needs of patients who do not wish to receive full disclosure, in such a way as to facilitate responsive, informed patient choice.

Euthanasia and end-of-life care

The ever-increasing capacity of contemporary medicine to extend life, regardless of the quality of that life, highlights a number of moral dilemmas and practical concerns that have been debated in professional and legal settings and in the mass media. Three dichotomies encapsulate these dilemmas.

- The sanctity of life versus the quality of that life
- Patient rights versus professional responsibilities
- 'Active' intervention versus 'passive' inaction

Euthanasia

Euthanasia is the act of intentionally bringing about another person's death for the sake of that person. Euthanasia is usually administered by a doctor and differs from physician-assisted suicide, where the person who dies causes their own death. A distinction is often made between 'passive' and 'active' euthanasia. *Passive euthanasia* is where patients are allowed to die and may involve withholding treatment or removing life support equipment. This is legal in Britain and other societies. *Active euthanasia* is where a person is helped to die by a physician. This is different from *physician-assisted suicide*, where a doctor helps the person to kill themselves (e.g. by providing lethal drugs). Another important distinction is between voluntary and involuntary euthanasia. In contemporary Britain it appears there is growing support for voluntary active euthanasia (i.e. at the patient's request) in clearly defined circumstances (e.g. intractable pain).

The debate about euthanasia in Britain has been shaped by the powerful lobby against it from the palliative care movement and by practice elsewhere, particularly in the Netherlands. Opponents of active euthanasia view it as a failure to provide good care whereas its proponents see it as allowing the assertion of personal control and individual choice. Personal beliefs about the sanctity of life are also important in shaping attitudes towards the acceptability of euthanasia.

After a long period when it had been practised under clear guidelines and protocols (Vander Veer 1999), voluntary active euthanasia was legalised for adults and children over 12 in the Netherlands in 2001, providing that:

- The request is voluntary and well-considered
- The patient is suffering from intolerable chronic pain

- The patient has a clear and correct understanding of their situation and prognosis
- A second doctor's opinion has been obtained
- Appropriate medical procedures are used to cause the death

Despite the social acceptance and availability of voluntary active euthanasia it accounts for only 2% of all deaths in the Netherlands. Some observers argue that the Dutch experience of euthanasia does not support the 'slippery slope' view that accepting active euthanasia will lead to the involuntary euthanasia (i.e. killing) of old and vulnerable people who do not want to die. However, the evidence is not conclusive and can be used to support both views!

The palliative care lobby argue that providing good palliative care, especially pain relief, will obviate the wish for euthanasia. However, results reported from a large national survey by Seale and Addington-Hall (1994) challenge this assertion. They report that about a quarter of both respondents and those who died felt that an earlier death would have been better and that 3.6% of those who died had asked for euthanasia at some point during their last year of life. The main reason for euthanasia requests appears to have been unacceptable levels of dependency, leading Seale and Addington-Hall (1994) to conclude that 'if good care is to obviate the desire to die sooner, it needs to address the problem of dependency as well as provide the symptom control in which hospice practitioners have developed such impressive expertise'. In a second paper (1995) they report that people dying from cancer who received hospice care were more likely to have requested euthanasia (8.8%) than those who did not (3.6%). It seems likely that hospice practices and philosophies that facilitate the expression of fears and encourage patients to exercise choice may explain this finding.

End-of-life care

Voluntary active euthanasia requires that the patient is able to express their wishes, usually when death is in prospect. Advance directives (or 'living wills') allow individuals to assert their preference to refuse life-saving treatment in specific circumstances *before* death is an imminent possibility. These originated in the US, where they have legal status. They have become increasingly common in contemporary Britain reflecting the wider societal emphasis upon individual autonomy and the right to choose (Chapter 10) and concerns about being kept alive by life support technology in a 'vegetative' state. Mass media reportage of high profile cases where the medical continuance of life has been challenged on the grounds of poor quality of life and the availability of proforma 'living wills' from organisations such as the Voluntary Euthanasia Society have also contributed to their increased use.

Although there is some confusion about the legal status of advance directives in Britain, a series of legal judgements in the 1990s led the BMA in 1999 to recognise that the oral or written advance refusal of life-saving treatments (e.g. cardiopulmonary resuscitation, CPR) is fundamentally the same as a patient's legal right to refuse other treatments. However, it argued that advance refusal of basic life-sustaining care (e.g. oral hydration and nutrition) should not be seen as binding.

There has also been concern about decisions made by health professionals not to resuscitate patients (DNR) for whom such action is deemed futile or detrimental to their quality of life (the ethical principle of malfeasance). Media reports of such decisions have suggested that they reflected ageism, and discriminated against older patients. They also seem to present an over-optimistic view of the success of CPR. Davey's (2001) study of an acute surgical unit found that communication between staff and with patients about DNR was poor and that patients' views were rarely sought (thus denying their autonomy). The ward nurses felt that rather than too many DNR orders there were in fact too few and often too late to protect their patients from futile and harmful CPR attempts. There was no direct evidence of ageism, although age was certainly a factor in arriving at a DNR decision.

The tension between the medical control of dying and the rights of dying people to exercise some control over decisions made about their treatment and death is likely to persist, but it seems unlikely that doctors and nurses will lose their central role in its management. Given the demographic composition of our society, the changing economic and social climate, increasing cultural diversity, advances in medical technology and a continuing emphasis on individual rights (Chapter 10), end-of-life issues will become harder to ignore and more difficult to resolve.

Summary

NHS hospitals remain the main places of death in British society, but most of the care of people who are dying takes place in their own home. Institutional care homes for the elderly have become more important as places where people live and die and the role of hospice and palliative care services is expected to expand further. Good end-of-life care in the twenty-first century will require better co-ordination between services to work across these settings. Nurses have an important role to play in such co-ordination as they are usually centrally involved in caring for those who are dying. Interpretations of how dying and bereavement are experienced have been framed in terms of the 'working through' of emotions in order to reach acceptance and adaptation to the death. However more recent models have questioned the validity of this framework for bereavement, recognising the continuing bonds that may be retained with the dead. As we move into the twenty-first century the wider societal pressures for greater patient involvement in the decisions about their end-of-life care will persist. The 'privileged' position of those dying from cancer is likely to be challenged and palliative care services extended to those with non-malignant chronic conditions. The need to respect the autonomy of patients from diverse cultural backgrounds is likely to become increasingly important, with more patients demanding consultation about resuscitation orders and the choice of euthanasia, while a sizeable minority may wish to remain minimally involved in such decisions.

References

Aries, P. (1983) *The Hour of our Death*. Peregrine Books, Aylesbury.

Copp, G. & Field, D. (2002) Open Awareness and Dying: The use of denial and acceptance as coping strategies by hospice patients. *Nursing Times Research*, **7**, 118–27.

Davey, B. (2001) Do-not-resuscitate decisions: too many, too few, too late? *Mortality*, **6**, 247–64.

Elias, N. (1985) *The Loneliness of the Dying*. Blackwell Publishers Ltd, Oxford.

Field, D. (1989) *Nursing the Dying*. Tavistock/Routledge, London.

Field, D. (1998) Special not different: General practitioners' accounts of their care of dying people. *Social Science and Medicine*, **46**, 1111–20.

Field, D. & Copp, G. (1999) Communication and awareness about dying in the 1990s. *Palliative Medicine*, **13**, 459–68.

Field, D. & Froggatt, K. (2003) Issues for palliative care in nursing and residential homes. In: *End of life in care homes: a palliative care approach* (eds J.T. Katz & S.M. Peace). Oxford University Press, Oxford.

Field, D., Hockey, J. & Small, N. (1997) Making sense of difference: Death, gender and ethnicity in modern Britain. In: *Death, Gender and Ethnicity* (eds D. Field, J. Hockey & N. Small). Routledge, London.

Firth, S. (2001) *Wider Horizons. Care of the Dying in a Multicultural Society*. National Council for Hospice and Specialist Palliative Care Services, London.

Glaser, B.G. & Strauss, A.L. (1965) *Awareness of Dying*. Aldine, Chicago.

Hinton, J. (1994) Can home care maintain an acceptable quality of life for patients with terminal cancer and their relatives? *Palliative Medicine*, **8**, 1834–96.

Katz, J.T. & Peace, S.M. (eds) (2003) *End of Life in Care Homes: a palliative care approach*. Oxford University Press, Oxford.

Klass, D., Silverman, P.R. & Nickman, L. (eds) (1996) *Continuing Bonds: New Understandings of Grief*. Taylor & Francis, London.

Kubler-Ross, E. (1970) *On Death and Dying*. Tavistock, London.

Lawton, J. (2000) *The Dying Process. Patients' experiences of palliative care*. Routledge, London.

Mellor, P. (1993) Death in high modernity: the contemporary presence and absence of death. In: *The Sociology of Death: theory, culture, practice* (ed. D. Clark). Blackwell, Oxford.

Parkes, C.M. (1996) *Bereavement: Studies of Grief in Adult Life*, 3rd edn. Routledge, London.

Payne, S., Horn, S. & Relf, M. (1999) *Loss and Bereavement*. Open University Press, Buckingham.

Riches, G. & Dawson, P. (2000) *An Intimate Loneliness. Supporting bereaved parents and children*. Open University Press, Buckingham.

Seale, C. & Addington-Hall, J. (1994) Euthanasia: Why people want to die earlier. *Social Science and Medicine*, **39**, 647–54.

Seale, C. & Addington-Hall, J. (1995) Euthanasia: The role of good care. *Social Science and Medicine*, **40**, 581–7.

Seymour, J. (2001) *Critical Moments – death and dying in intensive care*. Open University Press, Buckingham.

Sontag, S. (1989) *AIDS and its Metaphors*. Allen Lane, London.

Stroebe, M.S. & Shut, H. (1999) The Dual Process Model of coping with bereavement: rationale and description. *Death Studies*, **23**, 197–224.

Timmermans, S. (1994) Dying of awareness: the theory of awareness contexts. *Sociology of Health and Illness*, **16**, 322–39.

Turner, L. (2002) Bioethics and end-of-life care in multi-ethnic settings: cultural diversity in Canada and the USA. *Mortality*, **7**, 285–301.

Vachon, M.C.S. (1995) Staff stress in hospice/palliative care: a review. *Palliative Medicine*, **9**, 91–122.

Vander Veer, J.B. (1999) Euthanasia in the Netherlands. *Journal of the American College of Physicians*, **188**, 532–7.

Walter, T. (1994) *The Revival of Death*. Routledge, London.

Walter, T. (1999) On Bereavement. *The Culture of Grief*. Open University Press, Buckingham.

Worden, J.W. (1992) *Grief Counselling and Grief Therapy. A Handbook for the Mental Health Practitioner*, 2nd edn. Routledge, London.

Further reading

Clark, D. & Seymour, J. (1999) *Reflections on Palliative Care*. Open University Press, Buckingham.

Dickenson, D., Johnson, M. & Katz, J.S. (eds) (2000) *Death, Dying and Bereavement*, 2nd edn. Sage, London.

Walter, T. (1999) *On Bereavement. The Culture of Grief*. Open University Press, Buckingham.

Part IV

Health Care

Chapter 10
Health Care in Contemporary Britain

Patterns of health and disease and the organisation and delivery of health care do not exist in a vacuum but are shaped by wider social processes. Thus, to understand health care in contemporary Britain, some understanding of British society is necessary. The characteristics and problems of health care in Britain are best understood in terms of its history as a modern industrial society and the more recent shift to a 'post-modern' patterning of social relationships. The chapter will:

- Examine the changing social context of contemporary Britain
- Explain how the changing social context impacts on health care
- Discuss increasing pressures on the delivery of health care
- Discuss changing aspects of the British health care system at the start of the twenty-first century

Contemporary Britain

Halsey (2000) describes contemporary Britain as 'a highly privileged country by any standards of longevity, knowledge and income'. This section discusses a number of important social changes during the twentieth century, especially since the 1960s, that have profoundly affected our society and its patterns of health and health care. It examines the transformation of work and industry, the diversification of family and household patterns, and concludes by considering more recent social and cultural changes.

The transformation of work and industry

Sociologists use the term 'modern society' to refer to societies based upon the industrial production of goods through the use of factory-based machine technology, with the great majority of the population living in towns and cities. In such societies people's life experiences and attitudes are shaped by this industrial and urban base, the central role played by the nation state, the predominance of bureaucracy and the dominance of scientific thought and technology over religion and traditional practices in shaping ideas, beliefs and values. At the beginning of the twentieth century Britain was a modern industrial society with over three quarters of the population living in urban areas, mainly working in large-scale organisations such as factories and offices. At the centre of the economy were the 'heavy' industries such as mining, steel and shipping. Current patterns of social relationships and their relationship to health and the provision of health care (discussed in Part II) can be traced back to these patterns of social, economic and political organisation. For example, regions with previous concentrations of heavy industry (the North and Wales) still experience higher levels of unemployment and worse health than the more affluent (mainly southern) regions.

Over the century technological changes and the increasing openness of world markets led to the decline of Britain's industrial base. From the 1960s there was a growing shift from manufacturing to service industry, with the proportion of manual workers shrinking from three quarters of the labour force in 1900 to less than a third at the end of the century. Long-term employment with one firm or within one industry has become less common in all occupations with a pattern of employment punctuated by 'job breaks' and retraining for new occupations emerging in the 1990s. Alongside these processes, and as part of them, has been the expansion of the 'public sector', including such basic services as health care, education and other aspects of the welfare state.

Contemporary western societies have had high rates of immigration and in consequence are characterised by cultural diversity. In Britain most immigrants have come from its ex-colonies in the Caribbean, Indian subcontinent and Africa and from Europe (Chapter 4). Since the 1950s immigration to Britain has been encouraged for economic reasons to meet labour shortages and this is still the case at the start of the twenty-first century, although the range of migration now reflects the increasing 'globalisation' of the world. Minority ethnic groups are largely concentrated in the most urbanised areas of England, especially London, although different groups are found in different localities. At the start of the century the increasing numbers of 'asylum seekers' has become a contentious political topic.

Another feature has been the steady rise of female participation in the labour force. Demographic changes, especially the decline in birth rates and the shortage of young males entering the labour market meant the range of work open to women expanded, as has the feasibility of a woman pursuing a career. Related factors are rising levels of educational qualifications of young women leaving school and the upgrading of entry-level courses to degree level for the mainly female occupations in health care. Currently most adult women work, although many married women are part-time employees. Part-time work is particularly common in the service sector. The increasing demand for well-qualified female labour has led many employers to provide a range of perks and services such as crèche facilities, planned career breaks, job sharing and flexitime to attract mothers with young children to work for them. These changes in the labour market for women have implications for nursing as it faces increasing competition for its traditional source of (female) entrants (Chapter 12).

Disposable income and leisure time have increased as the nature of work has been transformed through developments in information technology, automation and the introduction of more flexible working. The twentieth century saw a general and appreciable rise in living standards over the century, substantial redistribution of wealth, and the introduction of occupational and state pensions reducing inequality in old age (Halsey 2000). Yet although household disposable income doubled in real terms from 1971 to 2001 inequalities in income and wealth increased over the last quarter of the twentieth century (Social Trends 2002) and Britain had the second largest income inequality (after the US) among western societies in 2001. There are continuing concerns about poverty and deprivation, although definitions of these have moved from the inability to meet minimum requirements for food, shelter and clothing to relative income levels and comparisons of the poorest to the richest sections of society (Social Trends 2002).

Diversification of family and household patterns

Values, beliefs and attitudes towards health and illness that shape personal hygiene, illness behaviour, lay remedies and attitudes to health professionals are learned in families. Family members often mediate between the sick and health professionals. At times of health and other crises, such as unemployment or bereavement, it is with family and kin that many people talk through their anxieties and seek – and receive – support.

At the start of the twentieth century two main types of family structures predominated. In some communities, especially those associated with working-class occupations where people worked and lived close to their place of work, patterns of extended kinship were common, although the extended family did not necessarily live together. Such family patterns can still be found. Elsewhere the 'nuclear family' of two parents and their children was the main household unit although the ties to their families of origin and other kin were unlikely to have been severed. Nuclear families became increasingly common with the decline of heavy industry and the development of light industry, increasing mobility of the population and increasing affluence. It is, however, a myth to think that the nuclear family still constitutes the typical British family (Allan & Crow 2001). In 2000, although just over half the adult population were married, only 18% of households were married couples with their dependent children and 12% were people living on their own (Living in Britain 2001). During the first part of the twentieth century families with many children were common. Throughout the century the trend was for a greater proportion of the population to get married, but from the 1970s this trend reversed and in 2000 barely half of those aged 18–49 were married. Families had fewer children and in 2001 the birth rate of 1.64 children per woman was the lowest recorded since records began in 1934. In 2000 almost two fifths of live births in Great Britain occurred outside marriage (Living in Britain 2001).

Current domestic and family life reflects the increasing fragmentation and fluidity of British social life, with a wide variety of 'family types', including same-sex households. Overall, families and households have become smaller, more fragmented and less communal. In addition to extended and nuclear families there are one-parent families, cohabitation without marriage and 'step-families', as well as increasing numbers of people who live on their own. These changes have implications for health and illness.

There has been an increase in the number and proportion of one-parent families (7% of households in 2000). These are typically headed by a woman and most commonly found in inner city areas. One-parent families have historically been associated with teenage illegitimacy and poverty and many of their health diffi-culties can be traced to the economic deprivation and hardships that most of them face. Dietary deficiencies, poor housing and environmental hazards often lead to injury (accidental and non-accidental), disease and psychological distress. Single parents are a disadvantaged group whose children are more vulnerable to illness. However, since the 1990s an increasing number of older, economically secure, single women have chosen to become single mothers. Also, an increasing number of extra-marital births are found among couples in a 'stable relationship' without marriage (although some may go on to marry). The rise in joint registration of extra-marital births (nearly 80% in 2000) suggests an increasing proportion of unmarried mothers have a close and continuing relationship with the father of their child and are members of households with regular incomes. This is reflected in infant mor-tality statistics. The lowest rates of infant deaths occur among babies born inside marriage, closely followed by those born outside marriage jointly registered by parents with the same address. The highest rates are for those born outside mar-riage registered by parents living at different addresses or by mothers living alone.

From the 1960s there has been a sharp increase in divorce and at the turn of the century Britain had the highest divorce rate in Europe, with 40% of marriages ending in divorce. Divorce is typically accompanied by remarriage or cohabitation (a pattern referred to as serial monogamy). Married people have lower levels of mortality and illness than divorced, widowed and single people, although most studies suggest that such benefits are greater for husbands than wives. For adults divorce may entail:

- Loss of emotional closeness
- Loss of social prestige
- Reduced economic resources
- Changed accommodation
- Loss of friendships
- Reduced contacts with children

The effects of divorce upon children appear to be variable although the immediate separation appears to be a time of profound emotional disturbance with long-lasting distress among a substantial minority of children.

Divorce and subsequent remarriage or cohabitation may result in complex family relationships and household structures. In 2000 step-families comprised just over a fifth of British households (Living in Britain 2001) and 10% of children were living in them. There may be ambiguities and tensions about social relationships within step-families arising from emotional commitments to members of previous family units. Continuing relationships (e.g. with grandparents) can be a source of tension and relationships with wider kin (e.g. old and new aunts and uncles) may be ambiguous. These issues may blur the responsibilities for the provision of lay health care and social support between step-family members. Although there is no evidence that modern families are abandoning their familial responsibilities of care, the reduction in family size and the fragmentation and complexity of modern family structures means that there are proportionately fewer people available to provide such care. Members of step-families, cohabiting couples or divorcees may feel less obliged to care for sick or aged relatives and ex-kin. The current pattern of deferral of child-bearing is likely to continue and, in interaction with the increasing involvement of women in the labour market, is likely to lead to a further reduction in the availability of unpaid lay carers.

Social and cultural changes

These changes in British economic and social life have been greatly influenced and shaped by the development of global labour markets and the growth of con-sumerism, most noticeably in the latter half of the twentieth century. These have been accompanied by other social transformations, leading some sociologists to argue that the nature of modern societies such as Britain is changing rapidly and giving rise to a profoundly different, 'post modern', pattern of social life (e.g. Giddens 1991; Beck 1992). In contemporary Britain the institutions which previously provided authoritative meaning, shape and coherence to social life such as the police, Christian churches, schools and the professions are less influential and previously fundamental and accepted social axes of social structure and self-identity such as social class, age and gender have become more fluid. These changes have been associated with the breaking down of old loyalties and patterns of behaviour and greater choice and freedom of action for individuals. For example, voting patterns have become less class-based; gender identities have become less rigid and less significant in shaping work and leisure activities; and cultural iden-tities based upon ethnicity are more prominent.

In terms of knowledge, the dominance of received truth, traditional, religious and scientific, has been challenged by easier public access to information and com-peting opinions, including access to competing ideas and explanations about health and illness. For example, in 2000 there were over 70 000 websites disseminating health information (Cline & Haynes 2001). Both scientific and religious knowledge may be challenged and found wanting. The rapid expansion of the availability of the Internet, mobile phones and other forms of 'instant communication' at a distance has, among other things, transformed the nature of time and space which now extend well beyond the immediate local setting. Indeed, the 'disembedding' of individuals from their localities is a key feature of 'post modernity' contributing to the greater choice and freedom of action for individuals and forcing them to become more self-aware in deciding their choice of behaviour (Giddens 1991). Thus, it is argued, the stability and persistence of institutions and lifestyles characteristic of previous eras is absent in post modern society, individuals' identities are less dependent upon their social backgrounds and social attributes (e.g. age or gender) and they feel freer to construct their identities through the lifestyle choices they make.

In terms of health behaviour and health care, this type of analysis may help to make sense of the growing emphasis upon individuals as consumers of health services and the commodification of such services through the introduction of market principles. It also partially explains the increased emphasis upon individuals taking responsibility for their own health and illness choices and increasing expectations of health care. However, a major difficulty in applying these ideas about 'post modern' societies to understanding health care and health behaviour is that they refer only to segments of society. While the globalisation, commodification and increased self-awareness affect all members of British society, it is the more affluent who are most likely (and able) to adopt 'post-modern' lifestyles. The poor, by virtue of their limited resources are locked into narrowly circumscribed local worlds and their possibility of making meaningful life choices are greatly restricted. Members of less privileged ethnic minority groups and the elderly are less likely to have access to such lifestyles than professional men and women. Thus, it is important to recognise that both the persistence of earlier patterns of social orga-nisation and beliefs and the fundamental 'post-modern' changes have implications for health and health care in contemporary Britain through the ways they shape people's lives.

Pressures on the NHS

The National Health Service (NHS) was conceived and initially implemented during and following World War II (Chapter 11). It aimed to provide a comprehensive health care service for all members of the society that was free at the point of access. In 1949 the NHS consumed under 4% of Britain's gross national product (GNP) or national wealth. Throughout its life it has expanded and consolidated its key role in British society. Despite fluctuations in the national economic fortune, since the 1960s around 6% of Britain's GNP has been spent on health services, less than other comparable countries, although this is planned to rise to bring Britain into line with other European Union countries (Figure 10.1; Chapter 11).

From the 1950s into the 1980s successive British governments struggled to control the costs of the NHS while remaining committed to the founding, egalitarian prin-ciples of providing a comprehensive health care service for all which is free at the point of access. During the 1980s the apparently irreversible rise in the cost of health care in Britain – as elsewhere – led to a fundamental reassessment of the organisation and funding of health care, leading to a more 'individualistic' and 'competitive' structure (Chapter 11) and eventually to increasing commercial involvement. A new consensus began emerging in the mid-1990s around a 'mixed economy' of health and welfare in which individuals and profit-making enterprises played an increased role alongside voluntary organisations and the State (Baggott 1998).

The founders of the NHS naively believed that its costs would stabilise once a pool of sickness had been 'mopped up'. However, its costs continued to increase above the rate of inflation and it is now accepted that the demand for health care is potentially limitless. Between 1977–78 and 2000–01 NHS spending doubled in real terms to £50 billion (Social Trends 2002) and the Wanless Report expected NHS spending to be £68 billion in 2002, projecting this to rise to £154–184 billion by 2022. Despite the continuing increase in government investment over its life, since the 1980s health professionals and others have been complaining that the lack of resources (including pay) and increased workloads are preventing the delivery of

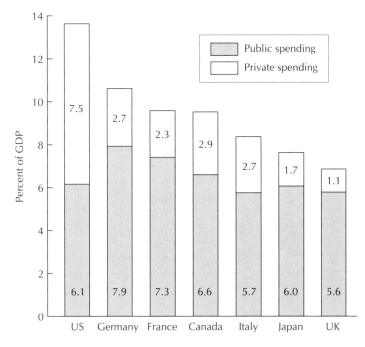

Fig. 10.1 Health expenditure by selected country. *Source:* Emmerson, C., Frayne, C. & Goodman, A. (2001) Should private medical insurance be subsidised? *Health Care UK*. Spring 2001. Reproduced with permission from the King's Fund, London.

high levels of care. However, when we look at the wider social context it appears that the problems of the NHS are due not only to 'under-resourcing' and deficiencies in its organisational structure but also to continuing external pressures on the service. Here we discuss four of these: Britain's ageing population, developments in medical technology, changes in the health care workforce and changing public expectations of health care (Figure 10.2).

An ageing population

A continuing pressure upon the NHS is the increasing numbers of older people in Britain. As discussed in Chapters 6 and 9 demographic changes have meant that many more people now live into old age than in earlier centuries and that older people now constitute a higher proportion of the population as a whole. In 2001 nearly a fifth of the population were pensioners with some 10 million people above retirement age. In 2000 7% of the population were over 75 (4.5% in 1971) and the number of over-85s continues to increase, projected to reach two million in 2020. Acute infectious diseases have been superseded by long-term chronic conditions as the major sources of illness and death in our society, and the burden of disease comes primarily from cancers and from long-term chronic conditions and their disabling effects (Chapter 7). These are conditions that primarily affect middle-aged and, especially, older adults. Almost 14% of adults living in domestic homes (as distinct from residential homes) have at least one disability.

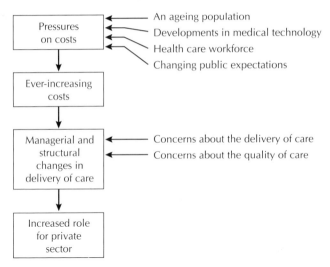

Fig. 10.2   Pressures on the NHS.

NHS expenditure per head is highest at birth and in old age (Figure 10.3). On average people aged 75–84 cost the health service more than four times the national average, with those over 85 nearly seven times more expensive. This, coupled with diminishing resources for lay care, has important implications for the health service. There are also significant costs to local authorities providing or paying for

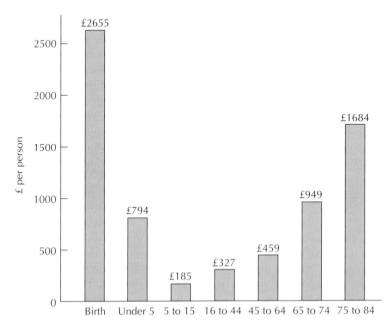

Fig. 10.3   NHS Health expenditure by age.
Source   Compendium of Health Statistics. Office of Health Economics (2002). Reproduced with permission from the Office of Health Economics.

statutory social services for old people, and to the families and 'lay carers' of sick and disabled old people. A common estimate is that the NHS requires an annual increase of 1% in its real income to keep pace with the additional costs resulting from the increasing number of old people in the population.

Medical technology

Within the medical sphere the continuing and seemingly ever-quickening pace of development of medical, surgical, and pharmacological technology have made new (and more expensive) forms of treatment possible, and led to more powerful and sophisticated interventions into matters of life and death. The development and marketing of new drugs increases costs in both hospitals and community general practice. Even technological developments which reduce the costs of treatment (e.g. by preventing heart disease or allowing day care treatment instead of hospitalisation) and initially reduce overall costs to the health service may in the long run increase overall health costs as simpler and cheaper treatments become more widely available, and more patients are treated. Developments in medical practice have therefore tended to increase health care costs. The Wanless Report (2002) estimated that medical technology adds between 2–3% a year to the growth in health spending. The establishment of the National Institute for Clinical Effectiveness in 2000 to scrutinise the effectiveness of clinical treatments was partly driven by the recognition that costly new treatments should be monitored for their 'cost-effectiveness' before being approved for general use.

At the same time that medical intervention has become more powerful, it has also become more complicated and dependent upon a growing range of specialists, thus making it more difficult to co-ordinate the various elements of treatment. The development of such techniques has been partly responsible both for the concentration of secondary medical practice in large general hospitals since the mid-1960s and the ever-increasing costs of hospital medicine. Advances in medical specialisation and high technology medicine have led to the development of a greater range of nurse and other paramedical specialists. This has altered the boundaries of nursing work, increased the demands on nursing staff and led to a greater range of skill mix in nursing care (Chapter 12). It also seems to have resulted in hospitals becoming primarily concerned with acute care with long-term care moving to other settings, such as nursing homes, which may be outside the NHS.

Changes in the health care workforce

Throughout its life the main cost for the NHS has been its workforce, accounting for over 60% of its budget. With over a million workers it is the largest employer in Britain. The costs of skilled staff in the NHS have historically risen faster than the general rate of inflation, adding about 2% above the rate of inflation to NHS costs (Wanless 2002). Health care is labour-intensive and government plans for improving the service have acknowledged that one of the main constraints upon delivering an improved service is the difficulty of recruiting staff at all levels. For example, the Cancer Plan explicitly acknowledges that improvements in cancer care depend upon the ability to recruit sufficient numbers of radiographers and specialist cancer nurses (Department of Health (DoH) 2000b). Significant expansion of the work-force is required if the government plans are to be achieved (Wanless 2002). The main difficulties in achieving such an expansion are:

- Increasing competition in the labour market, especially for more highly qualified workers
- Uncompetitive rates of pay and conditions of service
- The relatively long time-frame required to educate and train skilled staff

The expectations that staff hold about their pay and working conditions have altered significantly over the life of the NHS, with the long hours expected of, for example, nurses, junior doctors, and general practitioners no longer being accep-table. This is partly due to changing societal attitudes to the balance between work and leisure and family life. The increasing numbers of women occupying specialist positions also means that a greater proportion of health workers are taking career breaks in order to bring up their children than previously. In combination these two factors mean that greater numbers of staff are required to staff the service.

Public expectations of health care

The Wanless Report (2002) identified the expectations of patients and the general public of the health service as one of the 'drivers' of health costs. Ideas of what constitutes 'health' and illness have changed over time. For the majority of Britain's population good health has come to be seen as a right, rather than as a matter of social status or chance. Health expectations have risen with the general increase in standards of living and quality of life since the 1960s leading to more health-seeking behaviour (e.g. preventive screening) and higher expectations of the outcomes of care. Whereas the current older generations appear to have lower expectations of health and functioning, those born since the advent of the NHS expect better levels of health and demand more from the health services (Chapter 6). The introduction and success of the NHS has been a major factor leading to such raised expectations. Yet despite the well-publicised and real benefits to individual patients of procedures such as renal dialysis, hip replacement and cataract surgery, there is debate about the contributions changes in medical technology have made to the improved health and increased longevity of the British population since the establishment of the NHS (Chapter 2, Chapter 6).

Health care in contemporary Britain

Many of the difficulties of delivering comprehensive and universal health care in contemporary Britain are located not in the NHS itself but in the wider societal context within which it operates. The net effects of continuously increasing expectations of health care and ever-increasing costs of providing such health care means that the NHS requires more money each year simply to keep pace with the additional pressure being placed on it. It is these growing external pressures that help to explain the paradox of the British people paying more money each year for a health service that is thought to be less able to meet the demands placed upon it and whose health outcomes compare poorly to broadly similar countries (Wanless 2002). Partly as a response to these pressures and perceptions there have been some significant changes in the last two decades to the way in which health care is organised and delivered (discussed in Chapter 11). Here we consider five aspects of health care in twenty-first century Britain: the mixed economy of health care, hospital care, care in the community, challenges to medical authority and individual rights and responsibilities in health care.

The mixed economy of health care

The original philosophy behind the NHS was that health care should be provided by the state and that access to care should be determined by need, not ability to pay. However, although the NHS was the major source of health care, it was not the only source of such care with contributions coming from other statutory agencies (especially social services), charitable organisations, commercial organisations and lay care. During the latter part of the twentieth century the role of lay care in the community and of voluntary organisations came to be increasingly recognised and an increasing role for commercial enterprise encouraged. Perhaps the most significant change in the mixed economy of British health care was the latter.

In Britain and in many other western societies there has been a shift towards a greater 'market orientation' in the provision of health care. Markets are institutions in which people freely exchange commodities (goods and services) for money. Those on the political right believe that free market organisations are generally more efficient and give consumers more choice than centrally planned, state-run organisations. However, it has been claimed that these arguments do not apply to health care. First, a market system of health care, as in the USA, often fails to allocate adequate health care to those who are most in need of it – the poor and the elderly. Second, private health systems tend to be less efficient and have higher administrative costs than state-funded systems such as the NHS. Third, the consumers of health care do not have the expertise to make informed choices about their treatment and so inevitably rely heavily on the advice of professionals. Finally, under a market system people may be persuaded to undergo treatments that they do not need.

There has been increasing commercial involvement in health care in contemporary Britain since 1980. The Conservative governments of 1979–92 introduced a 'market orientation' into the provision of health care by introducing compulsory competitive tendering for ancillary services such as catering, cleaning and laundry. In 1979 private contractors undertook only 2% of NHS ancillary services. By 1985 the figure had risen to 40%, falling back to less than 25% following concerns about the quality of work and standards of hygiene, concerns that persist into the twenty-first century. Subsequent governments introduced and expanded Public Finance Initiatives under which companies contracted to provide facilities and services to NHS purchasers (Chapter 11). In 2002 the government reaffirmed its intention to use the private sector to work in conjunction with NHS services to expand capacity, increase access and promote diversity in the provision and choice of health services (DoH 2002). This approach has been resisted by health unions and other critics who regard the private sector as parasitical, making large profits at the expense of the public. Critics also fear that the continued growth of private sector involvement in the health service will further undermine the egalitarian principles upon which the NHS was founded.

Although there has been a substantial expansion of private sector health care, this accounted for only 16% of total spending on health care in 1998, significantly below that in other modern societies (Emmerson *et al.* 2001). Private sector involvement is much higher in areas such as non-acute surgery, long-term care of the elderly and reproductive medicine and many nurses are finding employment in nursing homes and other private sector institutions in preference to employment within the NHS. Around three quarters of all those using private health care outside the NHS pay for it with health insurance, usually purchased by their employers. The Wanless Report (2002) estimated private health insurance amounted to 1.2% of GNP. In 1971 2.1 million people had private health insurance, this increased rapidly during the 1980s reaching 6.9 million in 2000 (Social Trends 2002). The growth of private health insurance for individuals is explained partly by government initiatives to encourage private health insurance and partly by people's perceptions about failings of the NHS, such as long waiting lists. There appears to be a trend for more people to make 'one-off' payments for individual treatment episodes (e.g. cataract surgery) in order to avoid long waiting times.

Hospital care

Hospital care has been at the centre of the NHS since its inception, with over 60% of the NHS budget being spent on the hospital sector from the mid 1960s, peaking at 68% in 1972/73. The second half of the twentieth century saw 'a decline in the numbers of hospitals and hospital care yet increased rates of hospitalisation' (Armstrong 1998). A number of continuing concerns lead to a fundamental reappraisal of the current role of the hospital:

- The high costs of hospital care
- The increasing complexity of surgical and medical treatments
- Iatrogenic complications such as cross infection
- Negative physiological, psychological and social effects of long-term stays

At the start of the twenty-first century hospitals remain at the centre of the NHS although their organisation and pattern of work has changed. Economies of size and the increasing complexity of hospital care have led to decreasing numbers of hospital beds, the closure of smaller hospitals and the centralisation of services into larger hospitals with a greater range of specialist staff and equipment. Improved techniques, greater use of day care and out-patient clinics and the extension of hospital services into the community have reduced the time patients spend as in-patients (although there is concern that some in-patients are now discharged too soon). Thus, hospitals have been largely transformed into centres dealing mainly with acute care, with the rapid turnover of more patients through fewer beds. The three-tier pattern of care proposed in 1995 for cancer services (DoH 1995) has become the template for the treatment of other conditions. Centres of excellence with 'leading edge' technologies based in large specialist hospitals offer highly specialised interventions and the treatment of rare conditions; general hospitals with recognised specialist units manage common conditions; the care of chronically ill patients in the community is increasingly managed through hospital departments rather than by GPs and community nurses.

Like any organisations, hospital activities are underpinned by a number of beliefs about what is important and how work should be done. These are drawn mainly from the bio-medical model of disease (Chapter 2), reflecting the dominance of medical staff in patient care, and function to structure hospital work and staff–patient relations. However, although this bio-medical model remains important in shaping hospital work there have been attempts, especially by nursing and other paramedical staff, to supplement it with approaches that pay more attention to social and psychological aspects of patient care. Effective information and communication are central to patient management, patient well-being and clinical recovery, and improvements in this area are seen by government as central to increasing patient choice (DoH 2000a, 2002). Within hospitals, nurses are particularly well-located to contribute to effective communication with patients as they have most continuous contact with and knowledge of them and play a central role in co-ordinating the range of tasks and activities involved in clinical and care work. With the complexity of much clinical work and pressure on their beds there is ample scope for 'minor' bureaucratic errors to have negative consequences for patients and staff, a feature of hospital functioning that has received frequent 'bad press' in the media.

Care in the community

The 'mixed economy' of health care lies at the heart of health care provision in the community although the boundaries between statutory, voluntary and commercial providers of care, the responsibilities of these, and how they work with lay carers are not always clear. One of the main difficulties is articulating the contributions of various care providers. Within the health service the differing interests of hospital-based staff, primary care teams and institutional homes (most of which are commercially run) makes joint planning difficult. Both health and social services workers may be involved in the provision of care and there may be difficulties co-ordinating between them, especially for categories of patients such as the elderly and those with long-term disabilities where it is not clear which service is responsible for funding care. Such ambiguity has long been recognised as a serious detriment to effective and responsive care in the community and in 2002 the government published plans to break down barriers between heath and social care to create 'one care system' (DoH 2002). Voluntary groups contribute to community care and can make significant contributions to improving the lives of patients and their lay carers yet access to and liaison with them by lay and professional carers may be problematic.

The care of non-threatening acute and chronic conditions has always taken place primarily in the community managed by General Practitioners, community nurses or simply through self-care at home. Although the hospital remains the focus for acute interventions and the treatment of complex conditions there has been a progressive shift in the care of certain categories of people requiring long-term care to community settings. The movement to 'de-institutionalise' the care of people with learning difficulties in the 1960s spread to the care of the mentally ill, culminating in the closure of many long-term wards and institutions in the 1980s (Chapter 8). While these changes seem to have been largely based upon the view that care in the community was more appropriate for such people, governmental stress upon community care also seems to have been motivated by the view that it would be cheaper care. It was at least partly due to the high costs of hospital care for long-term conditions that care of people with physical disabilities and of the elderly in the community (e.g. in nursing homes) also became priorities, changing most hospitals into providers of acute care by the end of the twentieth century. More recently, the development of day surgery and 'hospital at home' initiatives has shifted some of the care of the acutely ill into the community.

While paid workers provide key elements of care *in* the community, the major source of care *by* the community is unpaid care from families, relatives and friends. This is often referred to as 'lay' or 'informal' care. During the 1990s the important role of unpaid lay carers in looking after chronically and terminally ill people (usually their relatives) in their own homes was increasingly recognised, with parliamentary legislation in 1995 establishing the provision of services to meet the needs of carers. The 2001 census found that there were over 5.8 million lay carers in Britain (almost one in ten of the population), a fifth of whom spent at least 50 hours a week on unpaid care. Older, chronically sick, terminally ill, physically handicapped and mentally ill people are particularly likely to receive lay care. Some of these suffer from long-term conditions and may be severely disabled, bedridden, incontinent or confused. Constant attention to therapeutic regimes and monitoring of symptoms may be required. Both men and women take part in lay care, although women are more likely to be the sole or main carer, to spend more than 20 hours in caring and to receive less outside help with their caring. A substantial proportion of carers are middle-aged, but a significant number are aged 65 or over, many looking after a spouse or very aged parent. Carers often experience a heavy round of daily tasks, a reduction in their social lives, and increased social isolation. They are frequently cut off from other carers and from the formal health care system. Financial costs may include job opportunities foregone by the carer (Maher & Green 2002).

Lay carers become eligible for their caring largely as a result of family ties and obligations. They typically have responsibility for most, or even all, aspects of their patients' welfare although they are rarely qualified or trained for their caring work. Lay care may be both open-ended and demanding and many carers are 'on call' at all hours of the day and night. Over a third of lay carers have no help with their caring work from others. The costs of care – financial, physical and emotional – to these lone carers may be considerable. Half of all carers have a longstanding illness themselves, and over a third (35%) rising to nearly a half (47%) among elderly carers, have limiting longstanding illnesses (Maher & Green 2002). There are few pressure groups to represent their interests or opportunities for them to meet others in like situations and the extent to which they are supported by professional workers varies, despite recognition that they are entitled to such support (James 1998).

Challenges to medical authority

Health care in western industrial societies has been dominated by medical science and the power of the medical profession. As near monopolisers of the right to treat the sick, doctors were in a very powerful position in their negotiations with the architects of the NHS and were able to extract a number of important concessions from the government, including the right to treat private patients. The final agreement between the government and the medical profession:

- Guaranteed the professional autonomy and clinical freedom of doctors
- Gave them a major voice in the allocation of health care resources
- Confirmed the power of the medical profession over other health workers, including nurses

During the 1990s challenges to this medical dominance increased. Perhaps most fundamentally the contribution of clinical medicine to improving health was questioned and a number of high profile scandals about medical mismanagement, failures and abuse of power eroded the trust of the lay public. Unevenness of care between different regions and hospitals are now well-publicised in a variety of government 'performance indicators', leading to questions about such apparent variations in the quality of care. Concern has been expressed that many contemporary interventions (e.g. screening for breast and prostate cancers) have not been subjected to adequate evaluation and may, in fact, be doing more harm than good by raising anxiety without offering effective treatment (Chapter 2).

Another challenge has come from other health professionals, including nurses. The medical profession has maintained its dominance over these groups through two main strategies. Some groups, such as nursing, have been subordinated to medical control and their activities largely delegated to them by doctors with little scope for autonomy, independence or self-regulation. This is particularly true in hospital settings, although medical control is lighter handed elsewhere. Other groups, such as dentists and pharmacists have had their activities limited to a specified range of activities, with the medical profession playing a key role in their registration procedures. However, nursing and other professions allied to medicine have successfully challenged the medical claim to exclusive expertise and over-riding competence as they sought greater autonomy in both their education and work practices, asserting their own areas of specialised skill and competency. Nursing has been aided in this by government initiatives to relieve the pressure of work on medical staff by reallocating clinical activities (e.g. prescribing, routine diagnostic procedures) and providing other sources of help and information to patients (e.g. NHS Direct).

The growing popularity of alternative or complementary therapies is another challenge to medical pre-eminence. Practitioners of 'alternative medicine' were for a long time excluded from the NHS, although they might be widely used within the community. In the mid 1980s it was estimated that these therapies involved about 6000 practitioners and were used by 1.5 million people annually, both of which have increased. By the turn of the century around a quarter to a fifth of the British population were estimated to have used some form of alternative/complementary medicine with similar or higher rates of use reported in western Europe and North America (Cant & Sharma, 1999). Alternative and complementary medicine are popular for a number of reasons.

- Their association for many people with a more 'natural' and 'holistic' approach to health and illness
- The failure of modern health care to offer effective and appropriate treatment for many chronic conditions
- The impersonal nature of high technology medicine and a desire for more patient-centred treatment
- Their contribution to a healthy lifestyle that maintains health rather than simply treating symptoms of illness

It should be noted that although a substantial minority seek help directly from non-orthodox practitioners (about a third of all users), most people using such practitioners continue to use conventional medicine, with many receiving con-current treatment for their condition within the NHS. An increasing number of doctors and nurses are taking such non-orthodox therapies seriously, with some GPs incorporating them into their practice. Osteopathy and acupuncture are now available to some NHS patients and other therapies are widely used in nursing homes and hospices. It is likely that alternative and complementary therapies will continue to be an important source of health care in twenty-first century Britain. However, Cant and Sharma (1999) argue that despite the 'limited legitimation' of some therapies and their apparent 'integration' into health care services this has not seriously threatened medical dominance.

The greatest challenge to medical power has come from government reforms of the NHS. The ever-increasing expenditure on the NHS led successive governments to attempt to make clinicians more accountable for the resources they used by imposing greater regulation, control and accountability upon doctors and other health workers. During the 1980s and 1990s the Conservative governments' strategy was to transfer power from the medical profession to managers. However, this managerialist approach appears to have been only partly successful in curbing medical power and control (Chapter 11). More recently Labour governments have adopted greater monitoring and more direct control of health professionals as part of structural reforms to the health services. This is combined with the claim that control of the NHS will be devolved from the centre to Primary Care Teams and hospitals, and that health professionals will be given greater discretion to make clinical judgements – *but only within the new systems of accountability and regulation* (Department of Health 2000a, 2002, my emphasis). The establishment of the National Institute for Clinical Excellence, the Commission for Health

Improvement and National Service Frameworks exemplify this attempt to shift power from the medical profession to government agencies through the greater regulation of their activities. Doctors and other health professionals have become more accountable to government for the resources they use and their clinical activities are more closely monitored than ever before.

Although real, these erosions of medical power have to be put into context. The British health system is still dominated by medical science and the bio-medical approach to treatment. Doctors, especially specialists, continue to enjoy considerable power, autonomy and status and to maintain their authority over other health workers. Medicine may be challenged but it is likely to retain its dominant position for the foreseeable future.

Individual rights and responsibilities

The growing emphasis upon the individual in contemporary Britain has led to an emphasis upon both the rights and responsibilities of individuals. The 1990s saw a growing concern within Britain for the rights of individuals to good standards of service and to clear information about goods and services. This has seen its expression in the growth of consumer organisations and an increasing propensity for litigation when expectations have not been met. Within health care, the concept of the rights of patients to minimum standards of service and informed choice was most clearly signalled by the introduction of the now defunct 'Patient's Charter' in 1991. In 2002 the commitment to patient rights was reaffirmed as a central aspect of the restructuring of the NHS (DoH 2002). At the local level providers of health services, such as NHS Hospital and Primary Care Trusts have been required to produce their own written standards. There has also been increasing openness with patients about diagnosis and prognosis. For example, many (but by no means all) patients have access to their own medical records (whether this improves clinical management of their conditions has yet to be established).

Patients have become more willing to challenge doctors' authority, with 95 994 written complaints about NHS services in England in 2000–01 (DoH 2001). While some welcome this trend as further evidence of patient autonomy in the face of the power of health professionals, the ethic of consumerism and the greater desire to litigate against doctors and nurses puts further strains upon a financially overstretched health service and those working in it (Chapter 12). In England around 10 000 new claims were made in 1999–2000 and the cost of outstanding claims amounted to £2.6 billion (National Audit Office 2001). The increasing propensity to sue health providers and the greater legal recognition of the rights of patients are factors contributing to the greater accountability of health professionals who now have to consult their 'clients' more fully and are less able to make decisions purely in terms of professional clinical criteria. The greater use of alternative or complementary therapies (noted above) and the apparently greater scepticism of medical science and technology can also be seen as part of the wider process of questioning and challenging scientific and expert authority.

While people have demanded and been given more rights, they have also been held more responsible for their own health. The major diseases of contemporary

British society are attributable to lifestyle and behaviour and the responsibility for maintaining health and preventing illness have become more explicitly defined by government and health professionals as the active responsibility of individuals. As discussed in Chapter 2, many areas of everyday life such as diet, alcohol consumption and exercise have become subject to medical intervention. The clients of medicine are no longer simply people who are ill, but potentially all of us, as witnessed by the health education and health promotion campaigns which exhort us to 'look after ourselves' to eat and drink 'sensibly', and to lead healthier lives. These developments are affecting the work of nurses and other health professionals, especially those working in the community, who are becoming increasingly involved with monitoring and regulating the lifestyle and behaviour of their clients e.g. the large amount of preventive screening work done by practice nurses.

Summary

This chapter began by looking at fundamental social changes in work and industry, family life and more recent 'post modern' social and cultural changes that have influenced the provision of health care in contemporary Britain. The predominance of chronic diseases, together with changes in family and household structures and in patterns of employment have placed pressures upon health services. Globalisation, increased access to information and greater freedom of choice have altered expectations of health and health-related behaviour. Demands upon the NHS are greater than ever before and the service is under continuing pressure from developments in medical technology and practice, rising consumer expectations and demands, and the costs of the health workforce. Changes in the management and organisational structure of the NHS have been made as a response to these continuing pressures, with fundamental restructuring promised into the early part of this century. One of the consequences of these changes is that the influence and control of doctors and other health workers is being challenged from a number of sources. Nurses entering the health service in the twenty-first century are entering a more diverse and fragmented set of work settings, including those in the private sector, with greater accountability for and auditing of their work than previous cohorts. However, whatever the organisational context of their work, and despite the increased importance of health promotion activities, the core of nursing – caring for sick people – is unlikely to change.

References

Allan, G. & Crow, G. (2001) *Families, Households and Society.* Palgrave, Basingstoke.

Armstrong, D. (1998) Decline of the hospital: reconstructing institutional dangers. *Sociology of Health and Illness*, **20**, 445–57.

Baggott, R. (1998) The politics of health reform in Britain: A Moving Consensus. In: *Sociological Perspectives on Health, Illness and Health Care* (eds D. Field & S. Taylor). Blackwell Science, Oxford.

Beck, U. (1992) *The Risk Society: Towards a new modernity.* Sage, London.

Cant, S. & Sharma, U. (1999) *A New Medical Pluralism? Alternative Medicine, Doctors, Patients and the State.* UCL Press, London.

Cline, R.J.W. & Haynes, K.M. (2001) Consumer health information seeking on the Internet: the state of the art. *Health Education Research,* **16**, 671–92.

Department of Health (1995) *A Policy Framework for Commissioning Cancer Services: A Report by the Expert Advisory Group on Cancer to the Chief Medical Officers of England and Wales* (Calman-Hine Report). Department of Health, London.

Department of Health (2000a) *The NHS Plan: a plan for investment, a plan for reform.* The Stationery Office, London.

Department of Health (2000b) *The NHS Cancer Plan: a plan for investment, a plan for reform.* The Stationery Office, London.

Department of Health (2001) *Handling complaints: monitoring the NHS complaints procedures. England, Financial Year 2000–01.* www.doh.gov.uk/nhscomplaints/background.html

Department of Health (2002) *Delivering the NHS Plan.* The Stationery Office, London.

Emmerson, C., Frayne, C. & Goodman, A. (2001) Should private medical insurance be subsidised? *Health Care UK,* Spring 2001, 49–65. King's Fund, London.

Giddens, A. (1991) *Modernity and Self Identity: Self and Society in the Late Modern Age.* Polity, Oxford.

Halsey, A.H. (2000) Twentieth century Britain. In: *Twentieth Century British Social Trends* (eds A.H. Halsey with J. Webb). Macmillan Press, London.

James, V. (1998) Unwaged Carers and the Provision of Health Care. In: *Sociological Perspectives on Health, Illness and Health Care* (eds D. Field & S. Taylor). Blackwell Science, Oxford.

Living in Britain. Results from the 2000 General Household Survey (2001). The Stationery Office, London.

Maher, J. & Green, H. (2002) *Carers 2000. Results from the carers module of the General Household Survey 2000.* The Stationery Office, London.

National Audit Office (2001) *Handling clinical negligence claims in England.* The Stationery Office, London.

Social Trends 2000 (2002). The Stationery Office, London.

Wanless, D. (2002) *Securing our Future Health: Taking a Long-Term View. Final Report.* HM Treasury, London.

Further reading

Halsey, A.H. with Webb, J. (eds) (2000) *Twentieth Century British Social Trends.* Macmillan Press, London.

Komaromy,l C. (ed.) (2001) *Dilemmas in UK Health Care.* Open University Press, Buckingham.

Chapter 11
Health Policy: Crisis and Reform

The previous chapters have shown that people's health, and their ability to cope with illness, are influenced by a range of social and cultural factors. This chapter considers another set of influences on health and illness, the impact of government health policy and of the kinds of health services that are available. As the provision of health care in contemporary Britain is the result of a long series of incremental changes and reforms, understanding health policy necessarily involves adopting an historical perspective. This chapter will:

- Define health policy and discuss its impact on health and illness
- Outline the development of the NHS and assess its strengths and limitations
- Discuss the major changes and reforms in health policy and the NHS in the 1980s and up to 1997
- Review the current Labour government's approach to health and assess the prospects for health policy and health work

Understanding health policy

Health policy is the term used to describe government decisions and actions aimed at maintaining and improving people's health. Health policy can include anything from a speech by a government health minister to a programme of legislation on health matters or, at the local level, the published goals of a health authority. However, it must include study of how well or badly policies have been *implemented* and what the final *outcomes* are. Policies are usually surrounded by conflicts over who is in control and how policies should be implemented. Therefore the study of health policy is concerned with the *political* and administrative dimensions involved in health and health care.

Health policy is a process of change and conflict: a policy cycle in which certain health issues come to the top of the political agenda (for instance, through media interest in 'health scares' or a health minister's interest in bringing about reform). These issues are either downplayed and sidetracked, or acted upon by government – with varying results in terms of implementation and outcomes (Figure 11.1).

Health policies are also shaped by 'external' factors such as the enormous cost of providing health services and revolutionary changes in medical technology and treatment (Chapter 10). Therefore, when looking at health policy in Britain or

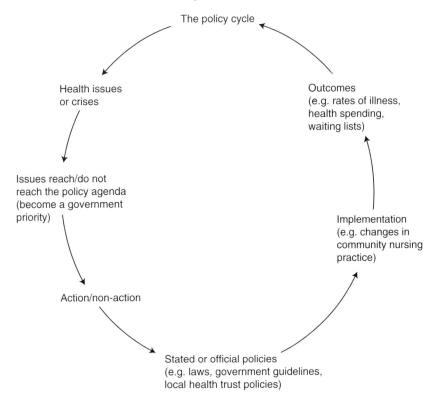

Fig. 11.1 The policy cycle.

elsewhere it is important to be aware that it is strongly influenced by factors beyond the control of governments. However, Figure 11.1 is useful in helping to think flexibly about the wide range of different government activities and policies which are directed towards health and illness – anything from a complete set of health reforms to a local anti-smoking campaign or new policies on nurse prescribing.

There are three kinds of government policy that affect people's health. First, there are policies on the health service itself, such as decisions about funding and running hospitals, primary care and community health services. These policies obviously have most direct impact on the working environments of nurses and other health professionals. Secondly, there are policies directed towards creating healthier environments (Chapter 2), such as those relating to the advertising and taxation of alcohol and tobacco, on health and safety at work, on environmental pollution and food standards and safety. Thirdly, there are government policies that can have a profound effect on people's health for better or worse, even though they are not specifically 'health policies'. These include policies on things like social security, taxation, housing and provision of social care. Although this chapter will focus primarily on policies concerning the provision of health care, it is important to remember that a wide range of other government policies also indirectly affect people's health.

The role of government in health policy

In Britain, as in most developed industrial societies, the government has come to accept increasing responsibilities for the health of its citizens – a reflection of a general development in modern societies in the twentieth century of widening state involvement in people's lives. It has been argued that the state's concern for the health and welfare of the population, and government provision of comprehensive health and social services, stemmed more or less inevitably from the gradual process of industrial and economic development. This argument suggests that industrial societies 'need' healthy, fit and productive workers and governments step in to meet these needs. However, there is no inevitability in the development of state-provided health services. The USA, for instance, is a highly developed industrial society in which health services have stayed largely in private hands. Although government in America plays an important part in subsidising certain health care costs and in regulating health care services, there is no equivalent in the USA of the kind of nationwide health policies or government health services found in the UK and other European countries (Stevens 2001). Thus the extent to which governments get involved in managing and providing health services varies significantly from country to country. There are also variations in the *range* of publicly provided services that are available, and in the *amount* of health care that the individual patient can be given through a state funded health service. Therefore, it is important to appreciate the distinctiveness of health policy in the UK. Britain was the first society in the western world to provide a state funded health care system that was free at the point of use for all its citizens. However, just as there was nothing inevitable about the development of a 'free' government health service in Britain, there is nothing inevitable about its continuation, at least in its present form.

Introduction and development of the NHS

The National Health Service Act (England and Wales) of 1946 aimed to introduce 'a comprehensive health service designed to secure improvement in the physical and mental health of the people ... and the prevention, diagnosis and treatment of illness' (Department of Health 1946). Before this, government responsibility (at local and national levels) for individuals' health and welfare was much more limited. There was no centralised, co-ordinated set of health services as there is today. For instance, before the NHS, hospital services were provided by a patchwork of voluntary (charitable) foundations, municipal (local government-run) hospitals, and private hospitals and clinics (Webster 1998).

   The NHS, which began treating patients in July 1948, was a landmark in health policy in two important ways. First, it was a centralised and government-dominated style of policy-making, despite the power of the medical profession to shape and alter policies locally. This traditional pattern of uniformity and control of the NHS by the Department of Health in London is now giving way to a less centralised approach – not least because of the introduction of devolved administrations in Northern Ireland, Scotland and Wales. However, compared with health systems in North America and in most European countries, it remains a uniquely uniform and centralised health service. Second, the introduction of the NHS represented a landmark because it was among the most socialistic and radical policies in the post-1945 Labour government's welfare state programme. The NHS formed a central pillar in the welfare state's ambition to provide equal care for everyone 'from the cradle to the grave'. However, the NHS not only represented fairness, equality and freedom from the worry of not being able to afford medical treatment, it also represented a turning point in policy about where the responsibility lay for people's health and health care. Along with the benefits of a 'free' National Health Service came the assumption that it was now primarily the *state's* responsibility to look after people and take responsibility for their health.

A product of conflict and compromise

Between 1946 and 1948, when the new health service was launched, there were fierce arguments between the government and the medical profession about how the NHS would be implemented and run. The NHS that emerged in July 1948 was the product of conflict and compromise. The government gained its objective of providing a new state health service for all, sweeping away the former distinctions between voluntary sector and municipal hospitals and establishing a service that would be 'free' at the point of use without any kind of means test. It was also successful in abolishing the pre-war system of state health insurance. After 1948, only a small fraction of the budget for the NHS would be paid out of National Insurance funds. Most of the funding for the NHS would be drawn from general taxation revenues, and this is still the case today.

However, the medical profession exacted a high price for its co-operation with the government. Before the NHS 'start date' of 5 July 1948 and as late as the spring of 1948, the British Medical Association (BMA) had threatened not to co-operate. A majority of doctors were worried about government control of their work and rates of remuneration. Consultants and senior hospital doctors were won over to the NHS in 1948 by 'stuffing their mouths with gold', as Aneurin Bevan – Minister of Health and architect of the NHS – put it. He was referring to consultants being allowed to treat private patients within the NHS and to the merit award scheme, devised to reward consultants for advances in medical treatment and research. Payment of merit awards represents a very substantial enhancement of consultants' salaries, and this practice was still in use in 2002, although there are proposals by the government to alter them. Family doctors were won over to the NHS by the government allowing them retain their independence as *contractors* to the NHS, paid on a 'capitation' basis; that is a fixed fee for every patient registered with their practice. This acted as a strong incentive to doctors to register as many NHS patients as possible, and to do so before rival doctors in their area signed them up. Doctors' representatives in both family practices and in hospitals were also very influential in determining how resources were to be distributed and over how their work for the NHS was to be managed. Thus although many doctors were initially opposed to state medicine, they quickly realised that the NHS *consolidated*, rather than compromised, medical power and autonomy. A major source of conflict in health policy in recent years has been between governments and the medical profession. Successive governments have initiated a number of reforms aimed at giving them more control over the NHS by curtailing the autonomy of health professionals in general and of doctors in particular (Chapter 10).

Evaluating the NHS

In many respects, making the NHS the centrepiece of health policy in the UK has proved to be a success. The NHS enshrines the laudable values of equality, fairness and compassion and, despite its acknowledged shortcomings, it remains popular with the public. Table 11.1 summarises the advantages and disadvantages of basing health policy on a comprehensive state-run service like the NHS.

Table 11.1   Evaluating the 'NHS approach' to health policy.

Advantages	Disadvantages
equality	uneven quality
access	referral problems
economy	under-investment
professionalism	waiting lists
	lack of accountability
	artificial divisions between services

Advantages of the NHS

Equality

The NHS was clearly an improvement on the inadequate and highly unequal jumble of hospital and family doctor services that existed before 1948 as it made access to both hospital and primary care available to all. It aimed to treat all patients equally, according to medical need, rather than perpetuating a health system in which the quality of services varied greatly according to where one lived. It also put equality before ability to pay for services. To its defenders this is a 'hallmark of a civilised society' when compared to the United States, where those without adequate health insurance are denied access to good quality health care.

Access

Because the NHS is based on a simple and effective principle of universal entitlement to health care, with no barrier of having to pay fees or prove insurance contributions, it has proved to be highly effective in terms of accessibility. Britain is also distinctive in having a comprehensive family doctor service that acts as a gateway to other services and effectively links patients to them. Many other health systems do not have a comprehensive medical service at the local community level, and access to primary care can be more difficult.

Economy

The administrative costs of the NHS are comparatively low compared to health systems that are based on private or social (state-organised) insurance schemes, thus leaving a higher proportion of the health budget for health care work. Having a centralised health service has also meant that national pay agreements could be agreed for the whole NHS. In less centralised health systems, local wage bargaining and competition for nursing and other medical staff tends to drive up the salaries of health service staff. Until recently, the UK spent significantly less of its national wealth on health services than the European norm (Chapter 10).

Professionalism rather than commercialisation

The principle of fee-for-service does not govern the transactions between NHS patients and health service staff as it does in private or insurance-based health care systems. Therefore, doctors, nurses and other health care practitioners are more likely to put their professional judgement of what the patient needs before any other considerations, such as a financial incentive to provide a range of treatments that are unnecessary.

The limitations of the NHS

Despite its many advantages, the NHS also has a number of 'design faults' that have resulted in it being in more or less continuous crisis since 1948. These problems have become particularly acute in the past few years. They can be summarised as follows.

Uneven quality of services

The 'NHS ideal' of equal treatment creates the impression that good quality health care is available to everyone, according to medical need and urgency. However, in practice, the quality of treatment people receive depends on where they live. Survival rates following treatment for cancer, for instance, vary widely from one area to another. A patient might be lucky to be referred to a consultant or a hospital where world-class treatment is available, or less lucky to be referred to other, second-rate facilities.

Referral problems

Although access to the NHS is extremely good in the sense that almost 100% of the population are registered with GPs, in practice the family doctor service can act as a barrier to other services. Instead of referring patients promptly for secondary health care or specialist services where needed, GPs can act as a delaying or filtering device. The capitation system (referred to earlier) means that the GP has already been paid to treat patients before they walk into the surgery. Thus unless the Department of Health provides specific financial incentives to GPs to meet certain targets, as it has started to do in a very limited way in the last ten years, there is little incentive to provide treatment or to investigate problems too deeply. On the contrary, there is an incentive to minimise the amount of time spent with the patient. This drawback in the GP service has been compounded by problems of poor communication, especially between GPs and certain groups of patients. Almost all older South Asian people, for instance, are registered with GPs but a significant number experience communication problems with their family doctors and sometimes find that their health problems are not being heard or attended to satisfactorily (Chapter 5).

Under-investment

The NHS provides a relatively low-cost health service. However, while this is an advantage to the taxpayer, and to governments anxious to control public expenditure increases, it is a significant drawback in terms of attempting to improve the quality of health care. While spending on the NHS has risen steadily during its 50-year history, it has not kept up with health spending in comparable industrial countries. By 1987, for example, the UK was still spending below 6% of Gross Domestic Product (GDP) on health. This compared with 11% in the USA, 9% in Sweden and Germany and 8% in France (Office of Health Economics 1989). More recently the government has decided on a sizeable increase in spending on the NHS, which is set to rise from 7.7% of GDP in 2002 to over 9% in 2008 (Blakemore 2003). The results of decades of limited spending on the NHS are now evident in long waiting lists, difficulties in obtaining and retaining nursing and other medical staff, and poorer treatment outcomes compared with other European countries. It will not be easy to reduce these problems even with the projected substantial increase in spending.

Waiting lists and delays

One of the main ways that the NHS has managed to hold down costs is by making patients wait for treatment. If the availability of facilities and medical staff expands relatively slowly and demand for 'free' health care expands much faster than supply, then a lengthening queue is the inevitable outcome. Waiting lists for medical treatment exist in other countries' health systems, but the NHS has experienced particularly marked difficulties in this respect. As a result, health care professionals in the UK often have to make difficult decisions about which patients are to be given priority. Thus, rather than providing universal health care, they are increasingly rationing it through the use of the waiting list (Klein *et al.* 1996).

Lack of accountability

There are growing signs of a crisis of confidence in the medical profession and of the NHS to monitor doctors' and nurses' work adequately, or to hold them accountable for negligence or malpractice. There has recently been a sharp rise in the number of patients claiming to have been harmed by faulty medical practice.

Medical negligence claims cost the NHS £3.9 billion in 2001 – double the cost in 1998 (Blakemore 2003). Also, the horrific case of Harold Shipman – a GP working in Hyde, near Manchester, who was found to have murdered 15 of his patients and is suspected of having murdered hundreds more – illustrated serious shortcomings in the system for checking medical practice.

Lack of accountability and weaknesses in the system of monitoring the work of the medical profession have also come to light in other circumstances – for instance, the case of systematic misdiagnosis of cervical cancer by James Elwood, a consultant at the Swindon and Marlborough NHS Trust (Blakemore 2003). The implications of these and other cases of malpractice and error are not that such problems are widespread in the NHS. The point is that these cases went undetected because the traditions of the NHS, which involved handing over to the medical profession much of the responsibility for running the service, encouraged a situation in which lack of accountability to the public or to external scrutiny could thrive.

Artificial divisions between services

The introduction of a unified National Health Service in 1948 offered an opportunity to integrate the services offered in hospitals with those at the local level (family doctor services) and in the community. However, by maintaining sharp distinctions between hospitals, GPs and community health services, the NHS perhaps exaggerated the importance of hospital care and missed the opportunity to invest more substantially than it did in family or preventive health services. Arguably, the NHS was from the beginning oriented towards becoming more a 'National Illness Service' or a 'National Hospital Service' rather than a *health* service. Similarly, there has long been a separation of health and nursing care from so-called 'social' care, or personal care of chronically ill or disabled people by non-medical care workers. As with the traditional distinctions between primary, secondary and public health services within the NHS, the health–social care distinction is now being questioned, and a great deal of health and social care policy has recently been concerned with trying to break down barriers to integrated care (Chapter 10).

Reform of the NHS

Faced with escalating demand for health care and limited supply of health care resources (Chapter 10), successive governments have initiated a number of reforms of the health service aimed at making it more efficient and cost effective in delivering high quality nursing care and medical services.

Conservative health reforms in the 1980s and 1990s

While the reforms of the 1970s were an attempt to make the 'old style' or 'traditional' NHS work in a more modern way by developing a more co-ordinated management structure, the Conservative governments' reforms of the 1980s and 1990s were far more radical.

While the Conservatives maintained the basic principles of a 'free' health service financed mainly by central government, they were determined to increase managerial control over health professionals and to make health care organisations more accountable for the resources they used (Baggott 1998a). These plans came to fruition in the NHS and Community Care Act 1990. The most radical reform was the introduction of a competitive structure into the NHS known as the internal market. This was based on the principle that money to pay for health services was supposed to 'follow the patient'. The NHS was divided into groups of 'purchasers' and 'providers' of health services. Health service providers, such as hospital trusts, were expected to compete against each other to provide their services to purchasing groups, such as health authorities and GP practices. The aim of the purchaser–provider split was to increase awareness of the cost of services and of improving efficiency. The more successful providers would attract more patients than the less efficient or cost-effective and efficiency was thus rewarded with more money and resources. There is little evidence that these reforms made the NHS more efficient, but they did bring about significant changes to the work environment of health professionals, particularly by undermining their autonomy and making them subject to more managerial control.

The Labour government elected in 1997 officially abolished the internal market in the NHS. However, a number of the fundamental features of the Conservative reforms are still in place and continue to influence the delivery of health care. Independent hospital trusts remain, the difference being that there is now less emphasis on market-like competition between service providers (though see the discussion of foundation hospitals below). Labour also widened the composition of primary care trusts, requiring more participation from representatives of professions allied to medicine, such as nursing and pharmacy, patients' groups and voluntary organisations. Labour has also retained the Conservative policy of apparently devolving more power and responsibility to local health service management while in practice centralising control over them by continually tightening targets and performance indicators. Those who run health services are allowed to meet targets in their own ways, yet face centrally imposed penalties if they fail.

Labour Government health reforms 1997–2002

Following the publication of various consultation documents between 1997 and 1999, the new Labour Government introduced a significant set of health policy reforms in the Health Act 1999. The main points of this, and subsequent, legislation can be summarised as follows.

Abolition of the internal market

The internal market in health care, and the distinctions between 'fund holding' and 'non-fund holding' GPs, were abolished. In England health services became administered locally by groups of doctors and nurses in primary care groups and trusts. These organisations manage the delivery of primary health care in their areas, chiefly through GP practices. They also 'commission' and plan other (mainly hospital-based) services for local patients. Thus primary care trusts control some of the resources available to NHS hospital trusts and to other providers, such as community health services (Klein 2001).

Integration of health and social care

The 1999 Health Act and the Health and Social Care Act 2001 both introduced reforms to integrate health and social care. The implementation of this is the responsibility of the primary care trusts, whose task it is to run health and social services jointly. In 2002 the formal integration of health and social care in a new NHS structure had not yet been implemented throughout Britain. However, early evaluation of pilot projects – for instance, a project to integrate mental health services in Somerset (see Blakemore 2003) – has shown that integrated care can produce marked service improvements for patients or service users.

Increasing central regulation and inspection of health services

The trend towards more centralised control of the health service is illustrated by the introduction of new government 'watchdog' organisations such as the National Institute for Clinical Excellence (NICE). This organisation decides which treatments, drugs and therapies are to be available to patients free of charge through the NHS. Another regulatory organisation, the Commission for Health Improvement (CHI), was introduced in order to inspect standards in primary health care and in hospitals. There are equivalent commissions to monitor and inspect social services and social care in each of the constituent countries of the UK. The CHI's work includes publication of 'league tables' of hospital trusts that include, for example, patient survival rates after various kinds of surgery and hospital treatment.

Increasing regulation of the medical and nursing professions

Some sociologists argue that one of the defining characteristics of contemporary societies is the increasing surveillance of people. We saw in Chapter 2 how an increasing number of nurses and other health professionals are now engaged in the surveillance of apparently healthy populations. Health professionals themselves are also under increasing surveillance as their performance at work is now subject to greater monitoring and control. The government introduced what are termed 'modern' contracts for GPs and hospital doctors. This policy is part of a drive to increase doctors' 'productivity' by making their pay conditional on reaching performance targets. This has met with some resistance from the medical profession. For instance in 2002, a significant number of hospital consultants and surgeons rejected government plans to link pay increases to a faster turnover of patients receiving operations.

The trend towards greater government control over nurses' day-to-day work can also be seen in a stream of new rules and requirements governing their tasks and responsibilities, working conditions, the quality of the equipment they are expected to use and the treatments they administer. Nurses' working contracts have been the subject of a number of government reviews. However, increasing accountability for nurses has been accompanied by increasing responsibility. A major policy document, *Making a Difference* (Department of Health 1999) established the government's commitment to extending the role of nurses, midwives and health visitors, and to developing a flexible training curriculum and, in 2002, the UKCC was replaced by the Nursing and Midwifery Council.

Thus while government policy has become increasingly concerned with delineating, specifying and scrutinising the tasks of nurses, doctors and other health practitioners, a contradictory trend in government policy has emphasised the importance of delegation of responsibility to 'front line' staff in the NHS. Nurses are expected to take more management and budgetary responsibilities, reflecting government belief in their importance for its 'modernisation agenda' for the NHS.

In sum, there are clear signs that the government wishes to introduce greater flexibility into the working practices of the different professional groups in the NHS. As part of this policy, it aims to rely increasingly on nurses to take over at least some of the managerial and medical work previously performed by doctors, or other health practitioners, or by health service managers. Whether this policy will lead to greater autonomy and a higher professional status for nurses, or to greater control and prescription of their work by central government, remains to be seen.

Preventive strategies in health policy

A distinct and interesting strand of Conservative health policy was a growing interest in public health and health promotion (Chapter 2). This change, and the government's strong endorsement of public health and preventative health care was something of a paradox. On the one hand, the Conservatives espoused the values of individualism, self-reliance and personal responsibility. On the other hand, the notion that there can be an economic payoff from preventative health policies must have acted as a strong appeal to their commitment to containing the spiralling costs of hospital services and other labour-intensive forms of health care. The result of these contradictions was a public health strategy that underplayed some of the more important determinants of health and illness (Department of Health 1992). Conservative policies on public health remained focused primarily on individual behaviour at the expense of tackling the social determinants of health and illness (Leathard 2000). For example, the well-established connection between poverty and illness was downplayed in *Health of the Nation* and other government policy documents. Addressing problems of poverty and of wider patterns of social inequality would have entailed a reversal of the government's strategy of reducing direct taxes on the incomes and wealth of rich and middle-income groups in society. Another limitation included a failure to ban tobacco advertising and sponsorship by tobacco companies of sporting activities (the latter issue also proved to be a sticking point in the succeeding Labour Government's health strategy). However, the Conservatives' drive to improve preventative health care contained a number of important initiatives such as action plans to reduce coronary heart disease and strokes, cancer, mental illness, HIV/AIDS and accidents. The government encouraged the development of 'healthy alliances', which were joint working groups (involving the media, schools, local authorities and employers) that were supposed to promote better understanding of health and to introduce healthier working practices. Thus issues of public health and of a preventative strategy were placed firmly on the agenda (see Leathard 2000).

In line with the history of the NHS, the new Labour Government's initial strategy to improve health is very much a hospital doctor, or health practitioner, focused strategy. Almost all the extra money spent on health is being used to improve curative services, and to try to bring the supply of complex medical equipment and of highly trained nurses and doctors up to the levels already provided in comparable European health services (Klein 2001). However, public health and preventative health strategies have not been completely neglected. In contrast to the previous Conservative administration, the Labour Government has explicitly recognised the connections between illness and low income, inadequate housing and hazardous environments. Labour's approach to public health was outlined in *Our Healthier Nation* (Department of Health 1998), a consultative Green Paper that identified the need to reduce health inequalities as a particularly urgent problem.

The strategies that have been employed by government to improve the health of people living in poorer and 'socially excluded' communities involve a bewildering variety of initiatives and schemes. For instance, a policy of developing Health Action Zones in a limited number of poorer communities and districts has resulted in the formation of partnerships between primary care trusts, local authority social services, private firms and local employers, schools and other education providers. These partnerships aim to develop awareness of 'healthy living' and provide opportunities to improve health in a variety of ways (e.g. improving diet, smoking cessation, awareness of drug misuse). Health promotion has been encouraged in local community settings such as nurseries and child-care facilities, schools and local colleges, and recreational centres.

Achieving change in health care

The Labour Government elected in 1997 initially tried to secure improvements in health services through further re-organisation rather than by significantly increasing resources (Department of Health 1997). However, the Labour administration that was elected in 2001 announced a substantial increase in public spending on health services (a third extra between 2001–06). It remains to be seen how far this increase will improve both service outcomes, such as reducing waiting lists or increasing number of operations performed, and improving people's health generally. According to the NHS Plan – the Government's list of objectives for the NHS that is updated regularly – the Government is expecting that its injection of additional money for health services in England will result, by 2006, in there being 20 000 more nurses, 2000 extra GPs, and 7500 more consultants. Over a longer period it is planned to build at least 100 new hospitals and provide 7000 additional hospital beds.

Despite claims by government that patients would soon begin to see marked improvements in health services, there are two main reasons to be cautious about the amount of improvement to be expected in the short term. First, in 2002 bottlenecks were already being experienced in attempts to increase the supply of nurses, doctors and other health workers. There are acute shortfalls in the supply of nursing and medical staff in all parts of the UK and additional staffing takes time to achieve. To cope with the shortage of nurses experienced in all parts of the UK, many health authorities are recruiting nursing staff from developing countries such as the Philippines and South Africa. However, doctors are more difficult to attract and the shortfall is likely to get worse before it gets better (Riddell 2001). Thus, after decades of restraining expenditure on, and staffing of, the NHS, and of following policies that encouraged health service managers to spread resources as thinly as possible, serious difficulties are being experienced in switching to a more expansionist policy.

A second reason to be cautious about the short-term impact of the Government's extra funding of health care is that strict conditions will be imposed on the release of additional spending. The Government made it clear that the extra money will only be released to health authorities or service providers where consistent improvements in performance are achieved. One of the main aims of Labour policy, as with the previous Government, is to increase central government control over health authorities and health professionals by having more inspection and more 'performance targets'. For instance the 'ten best' and 'ten worst' hospital trusts in England, evaluated in terms of their effectiveness in both providing treatments and in their use of resources, are to be identified each year. One drawback of this is that the system for monitoring performance and providing reports on quality may become an additional burden on nurses, doctors and other health service practitioners. Time spent by health professionals completing statistical returns and lengthy reports on their work means time taken from patient care. Also, while rewarding the better health service providers with the additional resources might have some justification in that efficiency is rewarded, it also means that resources are being withheld from the hospitals and other services that need them to improve. Thus, in the short run at least, this policy is likely to increase the existing unevenness in the quality of health services.

Another important part of the Government's policy, launched in 2002, was the creation of 'foundation hospitals'. The Government's chief aim in designating some hospitals as 'foundations' was to create centres of excellence that would act as examples of 'best practice' to surrounding hospital trusts. Foundation hospitals will continue to be public, NHS institutions but will be entirely self-governing and have the freedom to manage their own finances. For example, they will be allowed to raise additional funds by borrowing from banks or other financial institutions. They will also be free to enter into a wider range of contracts with the private sector of health services, and to negotiate their own pay rates for nurses, doctors and other health workers independently of national pay scales. Foundation hospitals have not been welcomed by everyone. There is concern that they will exacerbate the uneven quality of health care and may represent the beginning of a process of gradual privatisation of the more successful hospitals in the NHS. In 2002 it is too early to tell whether these fears will be justified as the development of the first 22 foundation hospitals in England has only just begun.

Private health care in Britain has grown considerably in the last twenty years, eroding the founding principle of the NHS that access to health care should be divorced from the ability to pay for it. First, the NHS has become more involved in the private health care market (Baggot 1998). Health trusts have developed marketing strategies to capture a growing number of private, fee-paying patients from private hospitals and, by 2000, they had won a fifth of the market share of private health care. Foundation hospitals are likely to stimulate even greater involvement of 'state' hospitals in the private health care market, especially as they will be able to attract the best and most able medical and nursing staff. Secondly, the private sector of health care outside the NHS has also grown considerably in the UK since 1980, partly through employers providing their employees with private health insurance cover. The proportions of the population covered by private health insurance vary widely around the UK, from a high of approximately 25% in the South-East of England to below 6% in Wales and the North of England.

Although no one can be certain about future trends in health care provision, it seems likely that reliance on private health insurance and private health care will continue to grow. The shortcomings of the NHS will act as a stimulus to better-off patients to obtain treatment that is quicker, and sometimes *perceived* to be of a better standard in a cleaner, safer hospital environment than in a standard NHS hospital. If this scenario of 'private options within an NHS framework' does develop, it is also likely to include other areas of health care than hospital treatment, such as additional nursing care or fast-track attention from GPs (Ham 1999).

Summary

Health policy can be defined as a wide range of goals and activities that mainly involve central government and that have a direct or indirect effect on health and illness. While some resources have been directed to preventative health care and public health since the development of a welfare state, governments, and the general public, have tended to associate 'health' with hospitals and medical treatments. The NHS provides a system of comprehensive health care available to all citizens and is relatively cost effective, but it also has a number of flaws in its design that have tended to obstruct attempts to make it more efficient and improve the quality of health care. Over the last three decades successive governments have tried to improve the efficiency of the NHS by increasing both managerial and centralised control over health professionals.

The Government has substantially increased spending on the NHS with the aim of improving the supply of medical facilities, nurses and doctors. However, progress may be slower than anticipated because of bottlenecks in the training system and the exit of qualified staff from the NHS. Dissatisfaction with NHS, particularly the time it takes to obtain treatment, has led to a growth in private treatment that is likely to continue in the foreseeable future.

References

Baggot, R. (1998) *Health and Health Care in Britain*, 2nd edn. Palgrave, London.

Baggot, R. (1998a) The politics of health care reform in Britain: a moving consensus. In: *Sociological Perspectives on Health, Illness and Health Care* (eds D. Field & S. Taylor). Blackwell Science, Oxford.

Blakemore, K. (2003) *Social Policy: An Introduction*, 2nd edn. Open University Press, Buckingham.

Department of Health (1946) *National Health Service Act (England and Wales)*. HMSO, London.

Department of Health (1992) *Health of the Nation*. Cmnd 1986. HMSO, London.

Department of Health (1997) *The New NHS: Modern, Dependable*. The Stationery Office, London.

Department of Health (1998) *Our Healthier Nation*. The Stationery Office, London.

Department of Health (1999) *Making a Difference: Strengthening the Nursing, Midwifery and Health Visiting Contribution to Health and Healthcare*. Department of Health, London.

Ham, C. (1999) *Health Policy in Britain*, 4th edn. Palgrave, Basingstoke.

Klein, R. (2001) *The New Politics of the NHS*, 4th edn. Pearson Education, Harlow.

Klein R., Day P. & Redmayne S. (1996) *Managing Scarcity: Priority Setting in the NHS*. Open University Press, Buckingham.

Leathard, A. (2000) *Health Care Provision: Past, Present and into the 21st Century*. Stanley Thornes, Cheltenham.

Office of Health Economics (1989) *Compendium of Health Statistics*, 7th edn. London.

Riddell, M. (2001) 'The New Statesman interview – Peter Morris'. In: *New Statesman*, 10 December, 20–21.

Stevens R. (2001) The evolution of health-care systems in the United States and the United Kingdom: similarities and differences. In: *Health and Disease: a reader*, 3rd edn. (eds B. Davey, A. Gray & C. Seale). Open University Press, Buckingham.

Webster C. (1998) *The National Health Service: a Political History*. Oxford University Press, Oxford.

Further reading

Blakemore, K. (2003) *Social Policy: An Introduction*, 2nd edn. Open University Press, Buckingham.

Leathard, A. (2000) *Health Care Provision: Past, Present and into the 21st Century*. Stanley Thornes, Cheltenham.

Chapter 12
The Division of Labour in Nursing

Chapter 11 outlined the key health policies which have shaped British health care over the last three decades. This chapter examines the implications for nursing of major changes in the organisation of the NHS such as changes in workforce planning. Breaking the boundaries between health care professions and developing flexible working practices so that the provision of care depends on staff skills rather than their job titles, are central to the government's 'modernisation agenda'. This has led to changes in the health care division of labour and the proliferation of new roles and specialties within nursing and at the start of the twenty-first century the content of nursing work is undergoing major changes presenting both opportunities and challenges for nurses. Following current conventions, the term nursing will be used to refer to nurses, midwives and health visitors unless otherwise specified. The chapter will:

- Discuss division of labour in health care
- Identify policies that have led to changes in the division of labour in nursing
- Discuss the difference between extended and expanded nursing roles
- Examine the experience of nursing roles and the new regulatory context

The division of labour in health care

The concept of the 'division of labour' – i.e. who does what – has a long history within sociology. It is associated with the nineteenth-century sociologist Durkheim (Chapter 1) who discussed the association between the division of labour between people and the nature of social bonds, or what he called social solidarity. In pre-industrial societies, common beliefs were strong and the division of labour between people was low. Since people performed many tasks in common, they were interchangeable in the division of labour. This meant that the loss of any one member did not pose a threat to the social solidarity of the community as a whole. As society modernised, the division of labour became more complex and specialised. Social solidarity now came from the differences, rather than similarities between people. Quite simply, as people developed different specialist skills, they came to depend more upon others. For example, when work is divided into a range of different tasks it is liable to break down if one of them is not performed properly. This was important for Durkheim because it showed that concerns about the increasing individualism of modern society were misplaced: far from being a threat to social solidarity, the interdependency that arose from the increasingly specialised division of labour meant that social bonds between individuals were tightening, rather than weakening. His work is important because it shows that individual autonomy is not a threat to the functioning of social groups.

Durkheim's insight is useful for understanding contemporary nursing work. The history of nursing is characterised by growing autonomy of practice as traditional hierarchies have slowly broken down both within the nursing profession and between nursing and medicine. As Durkheim might have predicted, individual autonomy has grown alongside an increasingly complex and specialised division of labour both within nursing and between nursing and other health care occupations. This means that even though individual nurses have greater autonomy in patient care than when nursing began, they also depend upon others more than ever before. The relationship between individual autonomy and interdependency is central to understanding the work of nurses in the health care division of labour.

The most important group that nurses work with is doctors, and the balance of power that favours doctors has a major influence upon their work. Freidson (1988) argued that the power of the medical profession had two interrelated dimensions: *autonomy*, or the ability to control its own work activities, and *dominance*, or control over the work of others in the division of labour. At the time he was writing doctors were usually able to make decisions about patient care free from external regulation by government and health care management. Patients were far less likely to question treatment decisions then than they are now, and nurses were largely cast in a 'handmaiden' role. For Freidson the professional dominance of medicine was problematic. Far from promoting social cohesion and contributing positively to patient care, it cast patients and other health care providers into subordinate and passive roles and inappropriately ruled alternative definitions of health, illness and approaches to health care out of consideration. In his view, the relationship between doctors and nurses (and doctors and patients) was characterised more by tension and conflict than by consensus and cohesion.

The subordination of nurses to the power of doctors in the division of labour has been an abiding concern of research from the 1960s onwards. In 1967, Stein suggested that the working relations between doctors and nurses were governed by the rules of an intricate game. He pointed out that doctors often found it difficult to maintain their confidence since their work is always to some degree uncertain and error prone. The cultivation of omniscience, that is of infinite knowledge and expertise, is a way of dealing with this. However, this omniscient status makes it very difficult for them to admit that they need nursing input in patient care. Even though nurses may have had greater knowledge and expertise than junior doctors, at the time Stein was writing they were discouraged from openly admitting this because of the prevailing norm of obedience to the medical profession. The twin factors of the omniscience of doctors and the subservience of nursing made it difficult for nurses to provide much input into clinical care, even though it was often needed, especially when junior doctors were unsure or made mistakes. The solution, according to Stein (1967), was the 'doctor–nurse game'. Each party is aware that the nurse is making a direct input, but neither directly admits to it. 'The cardinal rule of the game is that open disagreement between the players must be avoided at all costs. Thus the nurse must communicate her recommendations without appearing to make a recommendation statement. The physician, in requesting a recommendation from a nurse, must do so without appearing to be asking for it'.

Stein's work has been an important benchmark from which to gauge changes in the division of labour between medicine and nursing. There have been many changes since his first paper, with much more scope for negotiations in hospitals and primary care settings than 20 years ago. By the mid-1980s, nurses were expressing widespread dissatisfaction with relationships with doctors and developing strategies for greater autonomy from them. These included the development of an academic knowledge base distinct from medicine and developing partnerships with patients through new models of nursing such as the nursing process and subsequently primary nursing. In 1990, reflecting back on his analysis, Stein concluded that despite important changes such as increases in nursing autonomy, more women doctors, and the decreasing social status of the medical profession, the doctor–nurse game was still alive and well (although changes might be expected in the future). However, other research suggested that, if not dead, the doctor–nurse game has become more complex.

Hughes (1988), drawing upon research on Casualty Departments conducted in the 1970s, argued that nurses are not always subordinate to doctors. Nurse–doctor relationships are not homogenous but vary according to the situational context. Moreover, nurses do not always 'play the game', indeed in Casualty they often offered direct advice and, although less frequent, senior nurses openly challenged doctors' decisions and took control of patients themselves (usually when working with junior or overseas doctors). Svensson (1996) developed these ideas further, arguing that Stein's model regards nurses 'as essentially powerless and able to exert influence only through indirect, manipulative strategies which only serve to reinforce prevailing power relations'. He stresses that it is through negotiation on the ward and in other settings that decisions are made about the organisation of work such as who does what, what kinds of work should be done, and when.

Based on his research in a range of clinical areas in an urban general hospital between 1989 and 1993, Porter (1995) identified four kinds of nurse–doctor relations (Table 12.1). The first of these he termed *unmitigated subordination*. Here nurses adopt an unquestioned obedience to medical orders and have no direct input into medical decision making. The second is *informal covert decision making*, where statements that nurses make about patient care are co-opted by doctors as their own (this is akin to Stein's doctor–nurse game). Thirdly there is *informal overt decision making*. Here nurses have an involvement in patient care, but it is not officially sanctioned. This type of interaction involves nurses suggesting, even requesting, that doctors (usually juniors) initiate or change an aspect of patient care. The final type, *formal overt decision making*, which nurses typically shied away from, involves taking formally sanctioned independent decisions about patient care. Porter remarks that unmitigated subordination has declined over time. Informal covert decision making – the 'doctor–nurse game' – can be seen as a step towards nurse autonomy as nurse–doctor relations began to lose their authoritarian characteristics. This was being replaced by the now predominant form of

Table 12.1 Nurse–doctor relationships.

Type	Nurses' role	Doctors' role
Unmitigated subordination	Obey doctors' instructions	Take decisions Give orders
Informal covert decision making	Imply actions 'Steer' decisions	Take decisions 'Hear' suggestions
Informal overt decision making	Suggest actions Discuss decisions	Take decisions Discuss decisions
Formal covert decision making	Take decisions Negotiate joint decisions	Take decisions Negotiate joint decisions

Derived from   S. Porter (1995) *Nursing's Relationship with Medicine*. Avebury, Aldershot.

relationship which is informal overt decision making. At the time of Porter's research, formal overt decision making was uncommon, but nurse prescribing and other role changes mean this has become more common in contemporary nursing practice.

Health policy and the changing division of labour

There are two interrelated reasons for the move away from the 'unmitigated subordination' of nurses towards increasing autonomy: new government policies and professional developments within nursing. Together these changes have created greater opportunities for nurses to expand their area of influence and to exercise greater control over their work.

Government policies

The provision of timely, high quality health care to the population depends, amongst other things, on the right balance between public *demand* for services and the *supply* of staff to provide this service. Striking this balance is particularly difficult in health care where both financial and human resources are limited. The mismatch between supply and demand has become especially acute in recent years. Demand for health care has risen steadily since the inception of the NHS. This can be attributed to an ageing population, the development of medical technology, and rising public expectations (Chapter 10). At the same time, the NHS has experienced serious difficulties in providing the appropriate number of skilled staff to supply the service.

The Wanless Report (2002) on the resourcing of the NHS explained that the rate at which future activity can be expanded is determined by capacity within the system. It emphasised the need for a growth in spending, but also argued that spending alone is insufficient to resolve the mismatch between demand for and supply of services. Most importantly it also requires having sufficient numbers of staff with the right numbers of skills.

The nursing workforce

At the turn of the century, over a million people were employed in NHS hospital and community services in England, approximately 45% of whom were nurses. Department of Health figures for September 2001 reported there were nearly 459 000 nurses, midwives and health visitors (approximately 258 000 whole time equivalents), about three quarters of whom were qualified (DoH 2002a). These numbers are, however, insufficient to match NHS activity, especially given the current demands of clinical governance, reducing waiting times and the implementation of the National Service Frameworks (Wanless 2002). The commitment to increasing staff numbers outlined in the NHS Plan (DoH 2000a) has been difficult to achieve. Even though the number of nursing and midwifery students almost doubled from 1995–96 to 1999–2000, about a fifth leave during training and about one third of newly qualified nurses do not register to practice. Since 1997, the number of leavers has outstripped the number of entrants. The problems of retaining qualified staff are most severe in the inner cities, particularly London where turnover rates in some trusts range between 11% and 38% (Finlayson *et al.* 2002).

The nursing shortfall is being addressed in a number of ways, including recruiting overseas staff, retaining older staff, encouraging returners, providing more supportive working practices within the NHS and tackling discrimination. The Nursing and Midwifery Council (NMC) (2002) reports a rapid increase in the numbers of registrants with overseas qualifications. In 2002 over half of new entrants to the register (16 161) were from outside the UK, including 1091 from the European Union (EU). Over the four-year period 1998–2002, nurses from outside of the UK and EU rose rapidly from 3621 to 15 064, with the majority coming from the Philippines, South Africa, Australia and India. Nursing has an ageing workforce. In 1993 more than half of registered nurses were under the age of 40, whereas in 2002 over half of those on the register were over 40. One in four were over 50 and therefore eligible for early retirement (RCN 2002a). The NHS is developing a diverse range of initiatives to improve the quality of working lives, including family-friendly and flexible working practices. There is an expectation that these changes will not only help to retain older staff, but also encourage qualified nurses to return to employment (for example after raising a family).

There is also recognition that the NHS needs to tackle both indirect and direct discrimination by age, gender and 'race' in order to retain and develop an effective workforce. About 90% of nurses are women although the proportion of male nurses has increased since the 1990s. The NMC (2002) reported that over 10% of registered practitioners were male in 2002, compared to 8.5% in 1992. This is expected to rise, as 15% of student nurses are men. Importantly, men are over-represented in senior nursing grades. This may reflect direct discrimination insofar as men are more likely to be selected for promotion on the basis of sex, and/or indirect discrimination, since women are more likely to work part-time and to take career breaks which are disadvantageous to promotion and further training (Davies 1995). Ethnic minority nurses, who constituted about 12.5% of the nursing workforce in 2001 (DoH 2002a), face similar problems of discrimination. Culley (2001) summarises research evidence that suggests that nurses from ethnic minority groups are disadvantaged in three main ways. First, they are less likely to be appointed to senior posts. Second, they are more likely to be working in the less prestigious specialities. Finally, there is widespread racial harassment from patients and their colleagues. Equal opportunity policies have been largely ineffective in addressing these disadvantages.

This brief workforce analysis has highlighted the problems in providing the appropriate numbers of nursing staff to deliver the NHS Plan (DoH 2000a). However, numerical increases are not the only important change. Changes in the workforce composition, or skill mix, are also important. Britain, which has fewer doctors per head of the population than many other western countries, currently does not have enough doctors to deliver a comprehensive, high-quality service (Wanless 2002). Medical workforce capacity has also been affected by the reduction in doctors' working hours. The Wanless Report advised that skill mix changes can make an important contribution to the potential mismatch between the demand for doctors and their supply. In the most basic terms, the 'up-skilling' of nurses to take on clinical tasks that were once the province of doctors is a key solution to medical workforce problems. A more highly skilled, trained and flexible workforce is also expected to make a contribution to staffing problems within nursing.

Changes in skill mix and the wider development of inter-professional working are seen as important not only to resolving staff and skill shortages, but also to enhancing the quality of care and providing a more satisfied workforce. *A Health Service of All the Talents* (DoH 2000b) argues that workforce planning has actively inhibited interprofessional working and failed to support the creative use of staff skills. It states that health care providers should no longer be thought of in terms of 'different professional tribes' and calls for concerted action to develop more flexible working practices whereby the provision of care depends on the skills of staff rather than their job titles. Breaking the boundaries between professional groups – such as doctors and nurses – and developing flexible working have become new orthodoxies in health policy circles (Allen 2001) and are central to the 'modernisation agenda' being rolled out across the NHS.

Developments in primary care are an illustration of this. Practice nurses, health visitors and district nurses working within the primary care team are engaged in a diversity of new roles in the interstices of the traditional nursing and medical work. According to Peckham and Exworthy (2003) 'role delegation and substitution between and within professional groups is changing the face of inter-professional relations in primary care'. Nurse practitioners are increasingly taking on roles which include diagnosis, telephone advice, and home visits. This has been facilitated by the development of primary care teams, as well as more specific regulatory changes such as the introduction in 1994 of nurse prescribing and its subsequent extension. By 2001 more than 22 000 district nurses and health visitors had been trained to prescribe for minor ailments, minor injuries, health promotion, and palliative care (DoH 2002b). Extension of nursing work into the clinical area is most evident in nurse-led units such as NHS Walk-in Centres which offer primary care services without an appointment.

These changes in government policy are just one lever for change in nursing practice. In theory they open up the possibility for the flexible working practices and new nursing roles that contribute to increased autonomy of practice. Change has also been stimulated by developments within nursing.

Developments within nursing

Changes in the accountability and governance of nursing in the early 1990s have been described as a watershed development for nursing (RCN 2002a). Prior to the introduction of the UKCC *Scope of Professional Practice* in 1992, nurses needed to have extended role certificates signed by doctors before they undertook any work that was not included in their basic training. 'Scope' changed the professional agenda by disassociating the scope of practice from particular tasks, associating it instead with the knowledge and skills needed for safe and competent performance. There is no longer a list of tasks that a particular grade of nurse can or cannot perform and in early 2003 the range of grades were to be replaced by a competency-based structure (DoH 2002c). It is expected that a specified scope of practice will be associated with broad pay bands into which particular jobs will be placed based on the levels of knowledge and skill, responsibilities, and physical, mental or emotional effort that they involve.

'Scope' provided the opportunity for nurses to develop their practice in innovative ways. It also intensified debate around the distinction between *extended* and *expanded* roles, the merits of each, and their implications for both nursing practice and the development of the profession. Basically, extended roles refer to work that is delegated by doctors, that is, nurses taking on what has traditionally been doctors' work. Expanded roles refer to nurses retaining a distinctive nursing base of practice, but extending it to encompass new skills and responsibilities. The changing policy context and the distinction between extended and expanded roles revitalised and added urgency to longstanding discussions about the definition of nursing.

Defining nursing

Nursing knowledge and nursing practice have always been difficult to define. Indeed, in the mid-nineteenth century, Florence Nightingale commented that 'the elements of nursing are all but unknown'. As recently as 1999, the UKCC stated that 'a definition of nursing would be too restrictive for the profession' (cited in RCN 2002b). However, three years later The Royal College of Nursing (2002b) produced the following definition, emphasising both the ability of nurses to exercise clinical judgement and to be patient-centred in their work. Nursing is 'the use of clinical judgement and the provision of care to enable people to promote, improve, maintain, or recover health or, when death is inevitable, to die peacefully'.

It further stressed that nursing cannot be defined simply by the content of its work (e.g. by particular tasks). Rather, it is nursing's knowledge base that is central. The document from which this definition is taken highlights clinical judgement, and clinical decision-making, i.e. nurses' intellectual activity (the hallmarks of professional status). With its stress on holistic, patient-centred care *and* the use of clinical judgement, the RCN definition is broad enough to encompass both 'extended' and 'expanded' role definitions of nursing.

Changes in the boundaries of care between occupations tend to generate disputes over the 'ownership' of different areas of care. Not knowing what nursing is (and equally what it is not), makes it extremely difficult to protect and develop existing areas of expertise. It makes it difficult to resist the encroachment of other occupations into nursing's jurisdiction and to stand out against requests to take on work that has traditionally been the prerogative of others. The defining feature of a profession is generally considered to be its distinctive knowledge, based on credentials gained through advanced training. This distinctive knowledge is the basis for creating exclusive control over a particular area work. Doctors, for example, have traditionally been able to establish control over substantial areas of health care work by successfully claiming that they alone possess the expertise to exercise the clinical judgement that is intrinsic to diagnosis and treatment. This is one reason why the medical profession has resisted attempts to standardise care through the recent introduction of clinical guidelines into the NHS. Because nursing has struggled to establish a distinct knowledge base and area of expertise it has found it difficult to follow this professionalising strategy.

The launch of Project 2000 in 1987 was an attempt to deal with this by moving nurse education into higher education. This was underpinned by a new philosophy, which stressed nursing's unique contribution to patient care. Drawing upon academic disciplines such as psychology and sociology, the intention was to develop a knowledgeable workforce who were able to reflect critically upon their practice. Emphasis was placed upon patient-centred care, reflected in 'primary nursing', which involves allocating 24-hour responsibility for a patient to a trained nurse who plans and provides individually tailored care. However, this has proven extremely difficult to implement with the staff shortages described above. Consequently a modified 'team nursing' model has often been adopted, comprising a mixture of trained and untrained staff, support workers and students working in a team led by a qualified nurse who takes responsibility for the management and supervision of care (Allen 2001). In practical terms therefore, nursing's professionalising project has been limited by the constraints and changing demands of the work situation.

Extended and expanded roles

Government policies and the strategies of nurse leaders emphasise the increasingly autonomous role of nursing within the wider division of labour. This implies a marked shift away from unmitigated subordination towards informal overt and formal covert decision making (Table 12.1). However, there is often a large gap between policy and practice. Nurses work across different fields such as education, clinical practice, management, in a diversity of clinical areas and settings in primary and secondary care, and with a range of experience and expertise ranging from beginning to advanced practice. For example, the Chief Nursing Officer (DoH 2000a) identified 10 key roles for nurses:

- To order and diagnose investigations such as pathology tests and X-rays
- To make and receive referrals direct, say, to a therapist or pain consultant

- To admit and discharge patients for specified conditions and within agreed protocols
- To manage patient caseloads, say for diabetes or rheumatology
- To run clinics, say, for ophthalmology or dermatology
- To prescribe medicine and treatments
- To carry out a wide range of resuscitation procedures
- To perform minor surgery and out-patient procedures
- To triage patients to the most appropriate health personnel, using the latest IT
- To take a lead in the way local health services are organised and the way that they are run

There will be considerable variation in the way in which these and other roles are implemented. Nurses' everyday experience, including their level of autonomy, is therefore likely to be influenced by the ways in which new roles are developed in specific settings. Although in reality nursing work is likely to combine elements of both expanded and extended roles, as 'pure types' they are a useful way of thinking about the different directions in which new roles might develop and the tensions within them.

The work context

In the *extended* role, the new roles that nurses take on are delegated by doctors. This is a form of labour substitution. Doctors shed tasks which, for various reasons, they prefer not to perform. This may be because they are seen as mundane or uninteresting, keeping them from what is considered to be more important and exciting work. In this context, nurses take on a more technical role. In the extreme scenario, nursing work can involve moving from patient to patient performing a series of discrete tasks such as taking blood or siting intravenous lines. In some contexts, this can be the best way of 'getting through the work' and making sure that patient needs are met. However, critics of the extended role approach stress that it leads to the fragmentation of care and abandons nursing's caring role. This point can also apply to more advanced forms of practice such as clinical nurse specialists and nurse consultants which take nursing closer to medicine. From the *expanded* role perspective, nursing is inappropriately mimicking medicine and adopting a bio-medical model of practice (Chapter 2). It is argued instead that new role developments should be embedded within a holistic model of care. The new philosophy of nursing embodied in primary nursing is central to this.

Extended roles involve not only the delegation of doctors' work to nurses, but also the delegation of the work of trained to untrained nursing staff. Health care assistants (HCAs), who were introduced into the NHS in 1990, are expected to take on routine nursing work. Much of this involves basic patient care such as help with eating, bathing, and helping trained staff with, or personally undertaking, procedures such as basic observations. Tensions at the HCA/trained nurse boundary concern the lack of value that is placed on 'caring work'. HCAs report feeling devalued as professionals, something which is reflected in the lack of a career-structure (Thornley 2001). From the *expanded* role perspective, sloughing off the caring role to HCAs undermines trained nurses' ability to work effectively. Nursing work often involves the 'layering of conduct' (Latimer & Rafferty 1998) or 'strategic multi-tasking' (Allen 2001). Trained nurses often embed routine caring and 'housekeeping' work in their skilled work, for example bathing a patient as part of assessing skin care or tidying bed areas as they update patients charts. Allen (2001) argues that from a caring perspective this is a pragmatic use of time that can 'make a vital contribution to the maintenance of a safe environment for patients'. From this perspective caring work and clinical work are indivisible.

The occupational structure

There are different occupational structures associated with the pure types of extended and expanded roles. The *extended* role tends towards a hierarchical structure: HCAs are distinguished from trained nurses and basic grade nurses are marked out from those with higher training. A raft of senior or advanced roles – with a range of titles such as clinical nurse specialist, advanced nurse practitioner and nurse practitioner – have developed and nurses in these roles are generally agreed to be working at a higher level of practice (although exactly what this consists of is not clear). Through these developments nursing retains, and may even be intensifying, its hierarchical structure. This reflects recent changes within the medical profession which, in response to government attempts to curb spending and to regulate practice in light of high-profile failures such as the murders of patients by the GP Harold Shipman, has increasingly divided into a rank and file of practitioners and a disciplinary and managerial elite in an attempt to retain autonomy of practice. A hierarchical structure may benefit nursing by re-introducing the clear leadership structure at ward or unit level that was lost with the Griffiths reforms of the early 1980s (the introduction of nurse consultants and 'modern matrons' are examples of this). Conversely, it can be argued that this further divides the nursing profession along lines that mimic medicine and distances itself from patients.

The *expanded* role stresses teamwork rather than a hierarchy of individuals in roles with different levels of skill and status and emphasises partnerships with patients. Its philosophy of the nurse's role is as a teacher or facilitator, enabling patients to marshal their own healing resources in the belief that 'involving patients as partners in care increased their knowledge and control of their health' (Salvage 1992). In the current environment of the NHS where care is organised by specialism and staff shortages inhibit innovatory practice, the delivery of holistic patient care through a participatory model is something of a tall order. However, many nurses justify the expansion of nursing roles in exactly these terms (Latimer & Rafferty 1998).

Gender

It has long been recognised that gender ideologies are intrinsic to the health care division of labour. Traditionally nurses, who are predominantly female, have been the adjunct of doctors; the 'unacknowledged co-ordinators, the supporters, the moppers up of tears and fears' (Davies 2000). In trying to shed this role and image, contemporary nursing has been split between adopting the conventional definitions of professionalism (as embodied by medicine) or trying to develop its practice along other lines. Extended and expanded roles represent and draw upon these different approaches.

Extended roles are a route to nursing autonomy through inclusion within a bio-medical model of practice premised on personal autonomy and self-management, impartiality, and emotional distance (Davies 1995, 2000). In coming close to the bio-medical model of practice, extended roles are seen by Davies and others as inappropriately adopting a masculinist approach to practice. Davies argues that instead of seeking inclusion in the 'masculine model', nursing should seek to transcend it by adopting a model of nursing that positively values feminine traits. She encourages nurses to develop a 'new professionalism' which is shaped by gender and, among other things, recognises interdependence with others (colleagues and patients), has collective accountability for practice, an engaged and committed stance towards clients, and involves the investment of self in the clinical encounter. These are the values that underpin expanded roles and 'new nursing'. However, although the 'new nursing' may claim to be acting in the patient's best interest, this may mask other concerns. For example, Salvage (1992) suggests that primary nursing uses patient-centeredness as a platform upon which to build a new nursing knowledge that is distinct from medicine and that it is part of nursing's professionalising strategy.

New roles and the organisation of work

Sociological research on the nursing division of labour shows that how nurses negotiate their new roles and police the boundaries of their work within the wider division of labour and organisational constraints depends more upon pragmatic decisions about how to get their work done than upon the philosophical principles discussed above.

In her qualitative research in a district general hospital, Allen (2001) examines the division of nursing labour, highlighting the 'jurisdictional ambiguity' that has been created by the introduction of new roles and blurred boundaries within nursing and between medicine and nursing. Within nursing, the shared belief that 'hands-on' care is central to nursing work and 'knowing the patient' generated strains between the senior staff, whose work mainly focused on ward management and bureaucratic tasks ('paper work') and the staff nurses who were responsible for the care of the patients on the ward. However, the other demands upon staff nurses themselves meant they were not always able to engage in such work and that support staff (HCAs and auxiliaries) were involved more frequently in routine hands-on care. Allen concludes that the practical concerns of managing their work meant that there was considerable blurring of the nurse-support staff interface.

Allen found that although there were tensions between the devolution of doctors' work to nurses and the professional discourse of nursing stressing the re-integration of caring into the nursing role, the realignment of roles across the traditional medical–nursing boundary was taking place with very little explicit conflict. Nurses undertook what she calls purposive 'boundary blurring work' in order to improve the management of patient care. Examples of such boundary-blurring were giving intravenous fluids which were not written up on a patient's chart and requesting standard blood tests so that they were ready for phlebotomists and to ensure that tests were carried out on time. Nurses (especially the more experienced ones) would make their own judgements about a patient's condition and act upon it, for example, requesting a blood test if a patient looked anaemic. They would also work within the spirit of one rule, even if this meant breaking another. For example, giving a saline flush (not prescribed by a doctor) after prescribed IV antibiotics had been given.

Nurses took such decisions to work across the traditional medical–nursing divide to benefit patient care and to increase their autonomy of practice. In general, they found it easier to 'do doctors' work', rather than to negotiate it with them, leading Allen to suggest that in some contexts it is more appropriate to refer to the *non-negotiated*, rather than the negotiated order of practice. Such flexible working contributed to clinical effectiveness and she reports that the doctors recognised the skills of the nurses and were grateful when their initiatives eased the burden of work. Although doctors, nurses and support staff were concerned about risk management and the threat of litigation this did not stop them from blurring boundaries in order to complete the work of patient care. However, it is unsurprising that nurses were more likely to take such actions when working with a doctor they trusted.

The extent to which negotiation about roles is felt to be necessary and the manner in which it takes place seems to be strongly related to the organisational context of work and the demands of patient care. In the 'fast time frame' of the post-anaesthesia care unit (PACU) studied by Prowse and Allen (2002) medical and nursing tasks were overlapping and fluid, although there were legal boundaries preventing nurses from performing specialised activities such as tracheal intubation. PACU nurses had a wealth of experience that meant they were often more experienced and knowledgeable than junior doctors and, unlike the doctors, were always with the patient. They used the whole range of variations of the doctor–nurse game (Table 12.1) in their interactions with doctors to influence interventions and to improve patient outcome. In routine situations elements of Stein's (1967) doctor–nurse game and Porter's (1995) 'informal overt decision making' came into play, for example suggesting that a junior doctor ask for clarification about drug use from an anaesthetist. They were more likely to take on a directive role in emergency situations where unexpected, rapid, accelerating physiological change could result in death if not immediately corrected. In such situations nurses were likely to become assertive and might independently start procedures such as administering oxygen and IV fluids to ensure that a patient's condition was not compromised when doctors were busy in the operating theatre or anaesthetic room. Nurses might also challenge doctors' judgements. Prowse and Allen give the example of a nurse who judged a patient to be not as conscious post-operatively as he should have been, but where the doctor had failed to appreciate this. She therefore began to maintain his airway while the anaesthetist 'just stood there looking', before finally agreeing that the patient did need help with his breathing.

Like the PACU, Accident and Emergency departments are fast-paced and changing environments where nurses usually manage the flow of patients through them. Research by Annandale *et al.* (1999) suggests that uncertainty and unpredictability in the number and case mix of patients in these environments has a significant impact on the kinds of roles that nurses are prepared to undertake. This involved balancing the needs of the collectivity of patients against the needs of individual patients. Although doctors appreciated this, their focus was more often upon the individual patient they were dealing with at a specific point in time. Working as a team in order to cover each other's work with patients meant that the nurses' work often became fragmented and task-oriented. This was particularly the case when the mix of nursing grades and skills was weak. As has been found in studies of other clinical areas, the extent to which nurses were willing and able to undertake 'new roles' such as venepuncture, taking blood gases, inserting venflons and cannulae varied according to the 'busyness' of the unit. Contrasting strategies were employed. Nurses might decide to *do a task* such as taking blood or suturing in order to speed things up. Conversely, they might decide *not to do a task* when it was busy, falling back on more traditional nursing duties such as admitting patients and doing their basic observations. This made it difficult to know what nurses would, or would not, do at any one point in time which sometimes caused confusion and problems with continuity of care.

Risk and regulation

Nursing, like medicine, is becoming increasingly subject to government and managerial control (Chapter 10). New nursing roles are expected both to benefit patient care and to increase the autonomy of nurses and their job satisfaction. However, realising these objectives will vary according to the particular characteristics of the environments in which nurses work. The new roles will also be influenced by wider pressures which cut across all settings, nurses' perceptions of risk, and their attitudes to the increasing regulation of their work by government.

Nurses increasingly feel that they are working in a climate of risk and uncertainty (Annandale 2002). The individual accountability which enhances the professional standing of nurses as a *profession* can also make them feel *personally* very vulnerable. *The Scope of Professional Practice* (UKCC 1997) indicates that in taking on new roles, nurses must be aware of any limits in their competence and decline duties unless they are able to perform them in a safe and skilled manner. Although this is very clear in principle and can be seen as a positive development that acknowledges the professional standing of nursing, in practice it can be difficult to realise. These requirements appear to heighten the concerns of individual nurses about their personal accountability and about the level of support that they might receive from colleagues and employers if something goes wrong.

There is evidence of confusion about the management of accountability for the scope of new roles and the standards that apply to them. In civil law, legal action is directed against the NHS Trust or employer rather than the individual nurse or doctor, and the Trust bears financial responsibility for damages. The nurse, like the doctor, has a duty of care to use reasonable skill and care in their treatment of patients. This can be problematic when crossing the boundary from traditional nursing work into the medical domain since it is not readily apparent what standard the nurse will be held to. This is not the general standards of care expected of a nurse, but rather the standards that would be expected of the person, traditionally a doctor, undertaking the task concerned (Dowling *et al.* 2000). It is therefore important that the legal context of new roles are clearly thought through and that clear guidelines on accountability if anything goes wrong are developed.

Although nurses are individually accountable, they work in a complex division of labour involving other nurses, doctors, managers and patients. The actions of others can enhance or compromise their ability to fulfil their duty of care. The decisions to undertake or not to undertake an aspect of patient care are often influenced by the perceptions of others not only in terms of their skills and abilities, but also of the extent to which they can be trusted to support the nurse. Allen's research (2001) shows that this can influence the extent to which nurses are prepared to blur boundaries when working with doctors. Although many nurses feel that new roles benefit practice, they also report downward pressure from management to take on roles to solve staffing problems. In this context individual accountability can be perceived more as a management tool to shift responsibility on to the individual nurse and away from management, than as part of autonomous practice. The pressures from management and feelings of vulnerability that can arise from the dependency on others in the division of labour may lead nurses to feel that they have responsibility for their work, but have little control over it (Annandale 2002).

Nurses' willingness to take on new roles is also influenced by patient consumerism. There has been a rapid rise in complaints about health care in recent years with written complaints increasing by 10.9% between 1999–2000 and 2000–01 (Chapter 10). Although more of these complaints were against doctors (43 930) than nurses (19 020) (DoH 2001), and there is no evidence that nurses in new roles are more likely to make mistakes than doctors in the same role, this has done little to allay nurses' fears. Many nurses have mixed feelings about patient consumerism. They appreciate that patients want to know more and question more, but they may also experience the informed patient as a threat. Patients' increasing vigilance and lack of trust can feel like an attempt to 'catch nurses out' and hold them accountable when things go wrong, even when the nurse is not at fault. This sense of threat takes on particular significance when nurses do not feel supported by management.

These feelings can have an impact on nurses' willingness to undertake new roles. Annandale (2002) found that some nurses pulled back from undertaking some tasks because their confidence had been undermined by their perception that a patient or their relatives were likely to complain and they feared making a mistake. Nurses also reported the need to 'cover themselves' and to 'watch their back' all the time by, for example, constant checking and re-checking their work and making sure that everything was documented. Documentation is very important since it is proof in a court of law. However, nurses feel that it has become excessive, especially when 'every little thing' is written down, irrespective of its relevance for patient care. Moreover, time spent on 'paper work' is time away from patient care, and this can compromise care. Personal vulnerability can also influence nurses' interactions with patients. While it may prompt good practice such as making sure that patients and their relatives are fully informed, nurses may also shy away from giving information through fear of giving the wrong information, or because patients or relatives may misinterpret what they have said, with adverse consequences for the nurse. Annandale (2002) reports that 83% of the nurses and midwives in her study felt that their concern about legal accountability was influencing their communications in these ways.

Summary

Changes in the nursing division of labour have been influenced by labour shortages in nursing and medicine, the demands for an increasingly skilled NHS workforce, the shifting balance in nursing's relationship to medicine and the professionalising strategies of nursing. These have provided opportunities for nurses to increase their autonomy and control of their work. The route that nursing should take to achieve this ambition has been the source of some contention: should it accept work 'handed down' by the medical profession or create new roles firmly based on nursing expertise and principles? In contemporary Britain nurses work in a wide range of settings, in a variety of different roles. For this reason it seems likely that new nursing roles will emerge that embody *both* the development of new nursing roles *and* taking on 'medical' work. While changes in the division of labour in the contemporary health care workforce offer nurses the opportunity to extend the scope of their practice, to increase their influence in clinical and management areas, and to practice more autonomously, government attempts to monitor the quality of health care and to regulate the work of health professionals may sometimes work in the opposite direction. The result may be that although historically nursing work has become more self-directed, nurses may feel that they have less freedom and independence than previously.

References

Allen, D. (2001) *The Changing Shape of Nursing Practice.* Routledge, London.

Annandale, E. (2002) Working on the front-line: risk culture and nursing in the new NHS. In: *The Sociology of Health and Illness Reader* (eds S. Nettleton & U. Gustafsson). Polity Press, Cambridge.

Annandale, E., Clark, J. & Allen, E. (1999) Interprofessional working: an ethnographic case study of emergency health care. *Journal of Interprofessional Care*, **13**, 139–150.

Culley, L. (2001) Equal opportunities policies and nursing employment within the British National Health Service. *Journal of Advanced Nursing*, **33**, 130–137.

Davies, C. (1995) *Gender and the Professional Predicament in Nursing.* Open University Press, Buckingham.

Davies, C. (2000) Care and the transformation of professionalism. In: *Changing Practice in Health and Social Care* (eds C. Davies, L. Finlay & A. Bullman). Open University/Sage, London.

Department of Health (2000a) *The NHS Plan.* Cm 4818-1. Stationery Office, London.

Department of Health (2000b) *A Health Service of All the Talents: Developing the NHS Workforce.* Stationery Office, London.

Department of Health (2001) *Handling Complaints: Monitoring the NHS complaints pro-cedures, England. Financial year 2000–01*. Stationery Office, London.

Department of Health (2002a) NHS hospital and community health services non-medical staff in England: 1991–2001. *Statistical Bulletin*, February 2002. Department of Health, London.

Department of Health (2002b) *Extending Independent Nurse Prescribing within the NHS in England*. Department of Health, London.

Department of Health (2002c) *Agenda for Change*. Stationery Office, London.

Dowling, S., Martin, R., Skidmore, P., Doyal, L., Cameron, A. & Lloyd, S. (2000) Nurses taking on junior doctors' work: a confusion of accountability. In: *Changing Practice in Health and Social Care* (eds C. Davies, L. Finlay & A. Bullman). Open University/Sage, London.

Finlayson, B., Dixon, J., Meadows, S. & Blair G. (2002) Mind the gap: the extent of the NHS nursing shortage. *British Medical Journal*, **325**, 538–41.

Freidson, E. (1988 [1970]) *Profession of Medicine*. University of Chicago Press, London.

Hughes, D. (1988) When nurse knows best: some aspects of nurse–doctor interaction in a casualty department. *Sociology of Health and Illness*, **10**, 1–22.

Latimer, J. & Rafferty, A. M. (1998) *Extension and Expansion. Emergent Roles in Nursing and Health Visiting*. Department of Health Nursing Executive, London.

Nursing and Midwifery Council (NMC) (2002) *Statistical Analysis of the Register, 1st April 2001 to 31 March 2002*.

Peckham, S. & Exworthy, M. (2003) *Primary Care in the UK*. Palgrave, London.

Porter, S. (1995) *Nursing's Relationship with Medicine*. Avebury, Aldershot.

Prowse, M. & Allen, D. (2002) 'Routine' and 'emergency' in the PACU: shifting contexts of nurse–doctor interaction. In: *Nursing and the Division of Labour in Healthcare* (eds D. Allen, D. Hughes *et al.*). Palgrave, London.

Royal College of Nursing (RCN) (2002a) *Behind the Headlines. A Review of the UK Nursing Labour Market in 2001*. RCN, London.

Royal College of Nursing (2002b) *Defining Nursing*. RCN, London.

Salvage, J. (1992) The new nursing: empowering patients or empowering nurses? In: *Policy Issues in Nursing* (eds J. Robinson, A. Gray & R. Elkan). Open University Press, Buckingham.

Stein, L. (1967) The doctor–nurse game. *Archives of General Psychiatry*, **16**, 699–703.

Stein, L., Watts, D. & Howell, T. (1990) The doctor–nurse game revisited. *New England Journal of Medicine*, **322**, 546–9.

Svensson, R. (1996) The interplay between doctors and nurses: a negotiated order perspec-tive. *Sociology of Health and Illness*, **18**, 379–98.

Thornley C. (2001) Divisions in health-care labour In: *Dilemmas in UK Health Care*, 3rd edn. (ed. C. Komaromy). Open University Press, Buckingham.

UKCC (1997) *The Scope of Professional Practice*. UKCC, London.

Wanless, D. (2002) *Securing our Future Health: Taking a Long-Term View. Final Report*. HM Treasury, London.

Further reading

Allen, D. & Hughes, D. with S. Jordan, M. Prowse & S. Snelgrove (2002) *Nursing and the Division of Labour in Healthcare*. Palgrave, Basingstoke.

Davies, C., Finlay, L. & Bullman, A. (2000) (eds) *Changing Practice in Health and Social Care*. Open University/Sage, London.

Index